Rheumatology Practice in Occupational Therapy

Promoting Lifestyle Management

Edited by

Lynne Goodacre
Lancaster University,
Lancaster,
United Kingdom

Margaret McArthur
University of East Anglia,
Norwich,
United Kingdom

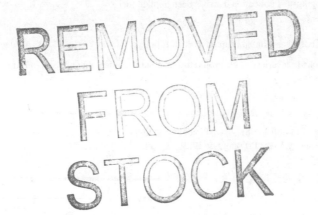
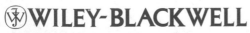

WILEY-BLACKWELL

A John Wiley & Sons, Ltd., Publication

Library of Congress Cataloging-in-Publication data has been applied for

ISBN: 9780470655160

A catalogue record for this book is available from the British Library.

Wiley also publishes its books in a variety of electronic formats. Some content that appears in print may not be available in electronic books.

Cover image: iStockphoto/CactuSoup
Cover design by Meaden Creative

Set in 10.5/12.5pt Times by SPi Publisher Services, Pondicherry, India
Printed and bound in Malaysia by Vivar Printing Sdn Bhd

1   2013

Contents

Notes on contributors

Jo Adams is Professional Lead for Occupational Therapy at the University of Southampton. She is an experienced musculoskeletal researcher and has a special interest in the clinical effectiveness of rehabilitation interventions.

Sarah Bradley is an Advanced Occupational Therapy Practitioner in Hand Therapy at Poole Hospital NHS Foundation Trust. She has over 20 years experience as an Occupational Therapist in hand therapy and has a special interest in the impact of rheumatic conditions in the hand and their therapeutic management.

Sarah Drake is a lecturer in Occupational Therapy at the University of East Anglia (UEA) specialising in psychology, sociology, occupational engagement and mental health. She has a special interest in predicting behaviour change, with a focus on factors that influence a person's intention to change.

Lynne Goodacre is an Occupational Therapist and Research Fellow at Lancaster University. She has worked clinically in rheumatology and the voluntary sector and developed a research programme exploring the experiences of living with and managing rheumatic conditions.

Alison Hammond is an Occupational Therapist and researcher at the University of Salford. She has particular interests in client education, joint protection, work rehabilitation, development of outcome measures and the evaluation of interventions through using clinical trials and mixed methods.

Janet Harkess is Head Occupational Therapist, Fife Rheumatic Diseases Unit. The Occupational Therapy service has provided a vocational rehabilitation service for the last 18 years.

Deborah Harrison is an Occupational Therapist is a lecturer at the University of East Anglia where she teaches psychology, mental health practice and qualitative research. She has extensive experience of working in mental health services.

Jill Jepson is a lecturer in occupational therapy at the University of East Anglia (UEA). She has worked in a variety of hospital, community and voluntary sector settings. Prior to joining UEA, she worked for the Bath Institute of Medical Engineering on assistive technology design and development.

Margaret McArthur is Director of the MSc pre-registration Occupational Therapy programme at the University of East Anglia. She has represented Occupational Therapy in a variety of profession-specific and other healthcare contexts. She has developed a programme of research related to management of change in long-term illness.

Lucy Reeve is an Occupational Therapist and works as a Specialist Lupus Practitioner at the Norfolk and Norwich University Hospital and as an Associate Tutor at the University of East Anglia.

Annette Sands is Therapy Lead at Wrightington, Wigan and Leigh NHS Foundation Trust. She is an Occupational Therapist with over 30 years experience of working in rheumatology and orthopaedics.

Penny Sloane is an Image Consultant and Personal Brand Coach. She is a qualified Master of the Federation of Image Professionals and a founder member of the Association of Stylists and Image Professionals.

Preface

The focus of this book is on locating occupational therapy interventions within the context of the personal experience of living with and managing a rheumatic condition. Our aim is to draw upon personal, clinical and theoretical perspectives to develop the reader's understanding not only of relevant clinical skills but of the clinical reasoning which is required to adapt and apply these skills within the context of individual client's experiences of living with a rheumatic condition. The book focuses on a person-centred approach and draws upon perspectives from occupational therapy, occupational science, health and social care policy, sociology and psychology.

We have spent a significant amount of time, within clinical and research contexts, listening to the personal narratives of people with rheumatic conditions who are trying to make sense of what is happening to them and to live their lives within the context of such challenges. This has introduced us to a different way of thinking about these conditions and what working in a truly person-centred way means. Many publications, by focusing on the development of clinical skills, lose sight of the challenges of integrating clinical approaches into the evolving context of people's lives. We suggest that this is fundamental to the ethos of the practice of occupational therapy and a central tenet of this book.

The first section of the book is designed to introduce readers to different perspectives of living with and managing a rheumatic condition, drawing upon the personal narratives of clients and therapists to explore these issues in detail. The importance of narrative is encompassed within the philosophy of occupational therapy where it is recognised that clients can be helped through the telling of stories. The first section also locates the management of rheumatic conditions within relevant theoretical and policy contexts shaping current approaches to the management of long-term conditions.

The second section of the book is focused on specific occupational therapy interventions with contributions. Throughout this section, each chapter provides insights into clinical reasoning and provides not only evidence-based information about the interventions but also the rationale behind their use. Contributors offer considerable experience in the management of long-term conditions, and many of the chapters are co-authored by an academic and clinical occupational therapist.

We hope that the book provides a unique mixture of personal narrative, theoretical perspectives and clinical skills appropriate to modern health and social care delivery which fosters a reflective critical approach in the reader.

Acknowledgements

Many people have informed the production of this book and helped to bring it to fruition. We would like to thank all of the contributors who have given freely of their time, expertise and experience.

Anyone working in clinical rheumatology will understand the sense of community which is derived from the multidisciplinary team ethos central to this specialty, and the same is true in the world of rheumatology research. Throughout our careers, we have been lucky to have learnt from many colleagues who have helped to develop our skills and expertise. We value greatly being part of this community and hope that in some small way this book makes a positive contribution to informing and developing current and future practice within this specialty.

However, it is the clients with whom we have worked, in both our clinical and academic lives, to whom we owe the greatest debt of gratitude. They have both informed our practice, challenged our thinking and opened up their homes and their lives to us, and it is to them that we dedicate this book.

Chapter 1

Living with a rheumatic disease: the personal perspective

Lynne Goodacre[1] and Margaret McArthur[2]

[1]Lancaster University, Lancaster, United Kingdom; [2]University of East Anglia, Norfolk, United Kingdom

1.1 Introduction

> Attention to human suffering means attention to stories, for the ill and their healers have many stories to tell.... The need to narrate the strange experience of illness is part of the very human need to be understood by others, to be in communication even if from the margins (Mattingly 1998, p. 1).

The aim of this chapter is to ensure that your focus is, from the outset, on the personal experience of living with a rheumatic condition illustrated by composite narratives informed by the many personal stories we have listened to and collected in the conduct of our research. We are conscious that in adopting this approach, we depart from the traditional structure of many clinical textbooks which usually start with an overview of the aetiology, pathology and clinical management of impairments. However, as suggested by Frank, 'not all stories are equal. The story of illness that trumps all others...is the medical narrative' (1995, p. 5). In a clinical textbook, it is easy for the clinical/medical narrative to dominate, and even though occupational therapy practice is informed by person-centred working, the voice of the person is often lost within the clinical story.

As occupational therapists who have worked clinically in rheumatology before moving into research, we are struck by the different narratives we hear when undertaking research to those we heard within our daily clinical practice. As researchers, we are alert to the emerging stories shared with us and those we work with are more obviously aware of their role as storyteller. Within our therapeutic encounters, some of these stories are unconscious revelations which still require due care and attention as highlighted by the following example. On a project looking at the social interaction of the client/practitioner

Rheumatology Practice in Occupational Therapy: Promoting Lifestyle Management, First Edition.
Edited by Lynne Goodacre and Margaret McArthur.
© 2013 John Wiley & Sons, Ltd. Published 2013 by John Wiley & Sons, Ltd.

relationship, there was an observation of a health professional taking the initial history of a woman who was being admitted to an inpatient rheumatology unit:

Interviewer, I; Hattie, H

I: Who is your next of kin?

H: Not my eldest daughter, she done my husband's funeral. She gets so terrible upset so she can't take no more.

I requests the name, address and telephone number of Hattie's younger daughter and it is supplied.

I: Would she be there at night if we ever needed to contact her?

H: They wouldn't have to get in touch with her would they?

I: No, it's only if there was an emergency, we need to have someone we can contact.

H: Because I don't get on with her husband you see.

I: No, it's only if there was an emergency.

—Hattie, 65 years, rheumatoid arthritis (RA)

Thus it is that in an effort to find out a factual piece of information (a contact telephone number), this person revealed information about:

• the death of her husband,
• problems experienced by her elder daughter and
• relationship problems with her son-in-law.

These issues were not acknowledged nor was an explanation given about what would constitute an emergency within the ward setting; however, the example serves to illustrate the centrality of narrative in our lives. Similarly, working alongside a client and asking a straightforward question can reveal how seemingly ordinary people have many stories to tell (Box 1.1).

Changes in healthcare delivery mean that there are far fewer opportunities for stories to be revealed in everyday therapeutic encounters. In a person's home, not necessarily being known as a healthcare professional, with more time to listen and a focus on understanding an experience as opposed to obtaining clinically relevant information, a different story is told that we wish to give voice to.

Narratives are described as collections of 'events, experiences and perceptions that are put together into a meaningful whole and understood/told as a story' (Goldstein et al. 2004, p. 119) and, when seen as a component of occupational therapy practice, through their telling, enable therapists to develop a greater understanding of people's worlds and experiences and how their lives are shaped by therapy (Mattingly 1998).

Narratives are constructed for an audience, they are told to people, and the way in which they are constructed and what is told is influenced by the audience. The clinical narrative recounted in textbooks is constructed primarily to educate healthcare professionals about the clinical management of rheumatic conditions, which by its nature seeks to address the problems and challenges with which people are faced. Within clinical practice, the personal narrative is often constrained by the structure imposed upon it by the questions posed; it is a guided narrative which seeks to convey specific information within limited time primarily focused on identifying issues to inform

Box 1.1

Betty came into the rheumatology inpatient unit, was assessed and treatment aims were established. She had to increase the range of movement and muscle strength of her shoulder, elbow, wrist and hand and improve her precision grip to increase her ability to perform personal care and writing tasks. Using the medium of batik, Betty produced a wall hanging depicting a tranquil scene of a church with a pond with ducks and bulrushes in front and a clear blue sky behind. The task fulfilled the aims of treatment, she gained satisfaction from completing each component part of the task and her function improved.

As part of the small talk that goes on in a treatment session, Betty was asked about her design. She began to talk about her childhood. She had been in Singapore during World War II and had been captured and placed in a camp. She spoke about how desperate life felt for her and how she retreated into her imagination of a scene very much like the picture she had produced in the treatment session. After talking for some time, Betty took stock of what she had been discussing and revealed that she had never told anyone about the image she had used. The aim of the session was to increase shoulder range of movement, increase stamina, and achieve the mindfulness of being absorbed in an activity with a view to increasing functional ability. What emerged as an extra dimension was Betty's need to tell her story about her childhood experiences. As Betty had revealed this aspect of her life, it was important to pursue it, offering other support services to allow her to explore this aspect of her life. On reflection, Betty decided that she felt at ease with the disclosure and had achieved enough by telling her story (Betty, 72 years, RA).

clinical interventions. However, these are partial narratives which focus on specific aspects of a person's life.

People participate in research for different reasons, but a common thread running through studies we have undertaken is the desire to give voice to an experience to enable others to understand. As suggested by Frank (1995), 'storytelling is *for* another just as much as it is for oneself'. In the reciprocity that is storytelling, the teller offers themselves as guide to the others. The resources listed at the end of this chapter illustrate how personal narratives have been used in this way.

When given the time and the opportunity to recount their story with little or no structure being imposed, the personal narrative assumes a different dimension in which illness is located within the much broader context of a person's life. At the end of conducting a research interview, it is common for people to comment that they have never had the opportunity to talk in such detail about their experiences before. The process of telling a story is one of making sense and giving meaning to an experience and has been used by researchers working within the social sciences to give voice to an alternative understanding of the experience of living with and managing long-term conditions, one grounded in personal experience (this work is explored further in Chapter 2).

1.2   Living with a rheumatic condition

The point at which occupational therapists come into contact with people with rheumatic conditions is often at the point in their illness trajectory when they are trying to make sense of what is happening to them. In Chapter 2, we will explore how this process is fundamentally about developing some kind of causal explanation. This is especially relevant to people who are often faced with medical uncertainty about the cause on their illness and seek to find an explanation for what is happening to them (Box 1.2).

Personal narratives also provide insights into how symptoms are labelled and categorised and how complaints are interpreted within a particular context or life situation (Kleinman 1988). For many people, obtaining a diagnosis can take time with symptoms being interpreted in different ways and even doubted by others until a definitive diagnosis is made, whilst others experience a rapid onset of their condition which turns their life upside down (Box 1.3).

Box 1.2

I work as a warehouse manager and have probably had AS for about 15 years or so but it's hard to tell really. It's only been diagnosed in the last 2 years. I've had back pain and pain in my neck and shoulders for years. At the time I put it down to the lifting and carrying I did at work and all the sport I played. I went to the doctors several times and was told I'd got a bit of lumber pain and to just get on with it basically so I put up with the pain on and off for years (Keith, 37 years, ankylosing spondylitis (AS)).

I keep trying to work out why it started when it did, as no one else in my family has it. All sorts of things go through your head. I remember having really bad flu and not really getting better very quickly but I can't really think of anything. Mum and dad hadn't been so good at the time and were needing a lot of support, and I was under a lot of stress trying to juggle looking after them and the family and my work; they say stress can be a cause don't they? (Sarah, 41 years, RA).

I have been a primary school teacher for 25 years. I hadn't been feeling well but thought it was because of the busy run up to Christmas. When I didn't feel any better after the Christmas holidays, I thought I had better see my GP. I am not sure he believed me at the start, probably thought 'oh here's another woman with a bit of a midlife crisis'. The back of my neck ached and felt stiff and it spread to my arms, hands and down my back; even my ribs and hips ache sometimes. I went to bed feeling tired and woke up even worse. The more tired I got, the worse the pain became. I started getting a lot of headaches and thought it might be eyestrain, so I went to the opticians but she said my eyes were good for my age! (Gemma, 50 years, fibromyalgia (FM)).

Box 1.3

About 2 years ago I got back pain which came on pretty quickly and didn't go away, and I just felt ill. Eventually, I went to my doctor's and she did an x-ray, but nothing showed up. Then she sent me for an MRI scan and I saw another doctor who told me it was ankylosing spondylitis. It was a relief after all these years to actually give it a name and know that something can be done (Keith, 37 years, AS).

At various points in time they have played with diagnoses of chronic fatigue syndrome, RA, lupus, depression and just back pain. My doctor did a load of tests and as each one came back negative he could tell me what I didn't have rather than what I did! He referred me to a rheumatologist who came up with the diagnosis of fibromyalgia; he pressed the places that were aching and they REALLY hurt (Gemma, 50 years, FM).

When I developed arthritis my daughter was literally a few weeks old; it just came on, all my joints were hot and swollen and painful, I was a mess. My parents lived close by and luckily had retired so were able to help otherwise I don't know how we would have coped. They were here every day. I couldn't pick her up, change her or feed her; you can imagine how I felt as a new mum having to watch someone else do all the things I had longed to do (Sally, 39 years, RA).

The variable nature of rheumatic conditions poses significant challenges affecting the ability to forward plan and commit to activities. It can also inhibit significantly people's social networks and social lives and impact upon their family life as flexibility has to be incorporated into people's lives. It also adds complexity to the maintenance of key roles, especially with regard to employment where people are required to accommodate variation into their working lives whilst continuing to undertake the requirements of their jobs (Box 1.4).

Alongside accommodating variability in the impairment, living with a rheumatic condition throws into uncertainty a person's ability to plan for their future.

> If it stays the way it is now I'm fine, but I do worry in case I'm going to get worse as I get older (Jo, 51 years, RA).

> I don't want to be self-employed and then this [RA] comes on again or everything stops working and I can't move and I have to quit, because I've got a mortgage (David, 37 years, RA).

Whilst previously people's perception of their future may have been associated with a deterioration in their condition, the recent introduction of anti-TNFα treatments has, for some people, opened up new possibilities.

Box 1.4

My lower back aches most of the time. If I don't keep on the move I can get pretty stiff. That's the trouble with having a desk job, but I suppose I'm lucky as I can walk around the warehouse. Sometimes it's worse than others; it's inexplicable really, there's no accounting for it. I can feel exceedingly tired and I don't know why that is. I might have a bad flare up for a week or so. Suddenly you can't walk without a lot of pain, you can't turn your head very easily and even turning in bed is difficult. I can't stand up to go to the toilet, and going downstairs is hard. I never understand why it comes and goes like this, and I've tried to work out if anything I do triggers it off (Paul, 39 years, AS).

I don't like being off work, I needed money, rents to pay, so while I was off work it did ease up [his symptoms], but when I had to give up work I was at my lowest point. I felt very depressed actually; I felt like it was a blow to the male ego (Colin, 55 years, AS).

It does stop you going out sometimes because if I was to fall over it I'd just be laying there because I couldn't get up and just the thought of something like that, little kids like they'll just laugh at you (David, 37 years, RA).

You just have to tackle a day at a time. You can't say to people, 'I'll do such and such with you' because you just don't know how you will feel until the day arrives (Brenda, 48 years, RA).

I stopped making any plans, you couldn't really plan or book anything to go and do, because you just didn't know you would feel OK (Mary, 62 years, RA).

My friend's daughter was getting married and I bought an outfit weeks before. On the Tuesday and Wednesday I had two really good days, but by the Friday I felt terrible, really awful and I thought, 'oh I'll just rest', you know, but I just couldn't go, I felt terrible on the Saturday and I just couldn't make it (Sally, 56 years, FM).

The pain you have to go through just getting up in the morning, just to try and put your shoes on, it's a bit of a nightmare (David, 37 years, RA).

I haven't got to worry about anything and I'm a man again because I'm earning, you see, it sounds daft but you like to be the provider, I used to hate sitting at home here and I'd be farting around hoovering and doing a bit of ironing knowing that the wife's been up since five in the morning, she's had to go to work and I felt pathetic (Colin, 55 years, (AS)).

[I can] take the children out for a day to a theme park, before I just used to be the bag person I looked after the bags, now, I can go on fairground rides, I don't have to think about it and I can enjoy it, it's like being a teenager all over again (Jane, 44 years, AS).

Although people on anti-TNFα often report feeling better, they do not necessarily experience complete recovery, 'I am just having a better life, I know my limitations they are not going to change' (Janet, 74 years, RA).

I had a year out of the gym, went back and I got a different programme. I don't do any classes now, I do Pilates, I can't really do them [the other classes] because anything with weights I can't put the weight on my wrists, it's all kind of saving them for the future. I need to keep my joints moving and everything, but anything that's more heavy impact can't really do, so even though I have gone back to the gym I still can't do the stuff that I used to do there's still a little bit of negative with it (Naomi, 20 years, RA).

The symptoms most commonly experienced by clients living with rheumatic conditions are pain, fatigue and stiffness (Box 1.5).

Whilst healthcare professionals often focus on the extent and duration of morning stiffness, clients will experience stiffness at different times of the day, especially if sustaining a fixed position for any period of time such as undertaking a long car journey or sitting at a computer for extended periods.

Box 1.5

Fatigue

My muscles ached and I felt constantly tired. I went to bed feeling tired and woke up even worse. People think I am just being lazy. The more tired I got, the worse the pain became (Gemma, 50 years, FM).

It's just that you're so much less of what you are because you just don't have the energy, probably people get a bit cheesed off or they do their own thing because you aren't there (Philip, 43 years, AS).

You sit at a bus stop and you're nodding and I fall asleep and that's what I call dangerously tired and that's bad because you can't keep your eyes open (Lily, 54 years, RA).

Pain

I seem to get really bad pain in my neck, like, real stiffness and when I went to the hospital last time he actually said, 'Well, don't paint the ceilings just concentrate on the skirting boards'. I did laugh but…that was one of sort of my main concerns, but then he laughed it off (Rob, 51 years, RA).

I was always in pain, always, it spoilt things for me and made life just pretty miserable (Alan, 56 years, AS).

Medical management

With the diagnosis of a long-term condition comes the need to engage with a range of healthcare professionals and to develop an understanding of the systems associated with the provision of health and social care. The majority of people will, for the first time, experience the need to take medication on a long-term basis, which, for many people, raises significant concerns:

> If I had my way I'd take none of them, it's all toxic no matter how good or how much it helps there's always a price for it, I haven't got the choice but if I had my way, if I thought I could get through it I would (Terry, 58 years, RA).

For some people, such choices are perceived in terms of a choice between quality or longevity of life:

> ...the issue I decided to take the drug on was quality of life, 'cause all these drugs shorten your life end of story, so the question is do you want to be old and crippled or do you want to die younger' (Sally, 56 years, RA).

Finding the right combination of medication can be seen as a process of trial and error with, over time, different medications and different combinations of medication being taken

Given the long-term nature of rheumatic conditions, the relationship developed with the healthcare team is often established on a long-term basis with, when it goes well, trust developing between the client and the members of the team.

> He's on my wave length that guy. I'm going places with my arthritis (Jo, 51 years, RA).

This relationship can, at times, be challenged when a person may feel at odds with the advice of the team and not want to put that relationship in jeopardy.

> I mean obviously if I do come off he has every right to say I told her to do it and she didn't so it's no wonder she's not getting better. I'd hate him to wash his hands of me cause I do like him and I trust him and I don't want to ruin all that (Lisa, 39 years, RA).

Challenges are not only posed by differing views about medication but also about other aspects of management such as engagement in exercises for people with AS. For clients and healthcare professionals, there is the need to establish an effective working relationship which recognises and respects an individual's right of choice and self-determination. Coming into ongoing contact with healthcare professionals requires people to develop an understanding of the nature of these relationships and responsibilities within them; people will have differing views about what these are:

> I think it is your responsibility to try and make yourself better. The medical profession can't offer you a cure so I think you need to do your bit as well (June, 45 years, RA).

The long-term engagement with healthcare services will potentially have benefits if there is a shared understanding and, therefore, an increasing familiarity with the expectations of the client, but the requirement to frequently retell the personal story can have negative effects as well:

This is so frustrating, relating my problems over and over again is emotionally draining, it's like facing up to it all over and over again. I just want to be pragmatic and get a solution not have to relive the nightmare of having RA again and again (Catherine, 43 years, RA).

Such emotions are often associated with completing official forms such as applications for welfare benefits which require a person to describe in detail the level of incapacity and activity limitation they experience.

Psychological impact

The variable nature of rheumatic conditions coupled with symptoms such as ongoing pain and fatigue and the impact of these impairments upon levels of activity can pose significant psychological challenges. Whilst, within a clinical context, attention can be focused on anxiety and depression, there are a wide range of challenges with which people are required to contend. Pain and fatigue can impact on levels of concentration:

Unfortunately I was unable to get much done and what I did do wasn't very good, I was just too tired to concentrate (Claire, 29 years, AS).

The inability to do things that had previously been taken for granted and the need to ask for assistance often cause high levels of frustration:

I sometimes think the frustrations worse than the disease at times. You get, I don't know about other people, but I get to tears sometimes because I'm so frustrated I desperately want to do something and just can't do it (Kate, 54 years, RA).

Activity limitation can lead to increasing work for other family members as they are required to undertake more tasks and feelings of guilt are often expressed due to this:

There are times when because you haven't done it, you know you're too tired or in pain, you feel guilty, really guilty and then your husband comes in from work and has to start preparing the meal or doing the ironing (Karen, 56 years, RA).

Some clients experience changes in their appearance, either due to the development of visible deformities, changes in gait and posture or the requirement to use appliances or dress differently to accommodate their impairment, all of which have the potential to mark them out as different:

Your self-esteem goes down sometimes. I mean you walk along the street and sometimes you get glanced at for your feet. I've heard people say I as they walk past me, 'did you see her shoes' (Brenda, 48 years, RA).

There can be an element of loneliness and isolation associated with living with a long-term condition highlighting the very personal nature of such an experience. Close friends and family develop an understanding of what is being experienced, but even on such a personal level there is a limit to how often they may be prepared to listen or a client feels able to discuss how they are feeling or the difficulties with which they are contending. Within a person's wider social context, there can be a feeling that such issues need to be concealed to reduce the impact of an impairment on the friendship:

> It's far more difficult to keep a friendship going because if you bug them with how ill you feel they are just going to go away, they're not going to put up with it. So there's no point in telling them how you really are. So there's a pretence that goes on you know, 'I'm fine thank you', when you're not fine, if you talked about it endlessly they'd just think, 'Oh it's her again' (Rebecca, 42 years, (FM)).

The accumulated impact of all of these factors accompanied by ongoing levels of pain and fatigue can, for some people, lead to periods of clinical depression:

> It's easy to say 'I'm depressed', because everyone does don't they but I mean it's that sort of, you know, where I want to sit and not move a muscle or not do anything whatsoever. But I do get up and I just go from one television to another and think, 'ee there's got to be more than this' (Linda, 61 years, RA).

> He said he was sorry I had lost my job but perhaps it was for the best. Which I thought was an absolute load of rubbish because I was very bitter about it and I was very depressed about it (June, 56 years, RA).

As well as the psychological impact of living with a rheumatic condition, when located within the wider context of people's lives, it is common for people to describe how stress related to another aspect of their life impacts upon their impairment, especially with regard to increased pain and fatigue:

> It's been bad for a few weeks and I went to see the doctor, but I think it was because I was worrying about my husband, he has been so ill (Mary, 53 years, RA).

Given the long-term nature of rheumatic conditions, over time people develop a repertoire of strategies to minimise the impact of the impairment on their lives.

1.3   Developing new skills and learning

As people live with an impairment, they develop a repertoire of skills and expertise which enable them, to varying degrees, to manage their impairment and the impact it has on their lives. Many of the chapters in this book provide detailed insights into the role of occupational therapists in facilitating this process with a specific emphasis on managing the symptoms and maintaining independence. In this section, we wish to draw attention to some of the wider challenges people face when locating the management of their impairment within the wider context of their lives.

A challenge of living with a long-term condition associated with change is one of adapting to each period of change as it occurs. Over time, people's accumulated experience of living with and managing a rheumatic condition becomes situated in their prior learning and informed by their past experiences (Box 1.6).

People accumulate and obtain knowledge from a wide range of sources, including self-help forums, the internet and a wide range of social media. Accessing such resources

Box 1.6

I have to have my full lunch break; my boss would let me work through if I wanted to and pay me for it, but I have to have time away from the (sewing) machines; I know if I push myself too hard, I will suffer at the end of the day (Jo, 48 years, FM).

I do still get these horrible tired feelings but I give into them easier now. I used to push myself and make myself carry on but now I can say, 'right you're tired sit down' (June, 45 years, RA).

If I'm in a lot of pain I will have a warm bath and put in a little bit of oil of comfrey or lavender and just rub where I am aching, and then have a warm drink and I've got an electric blanket, and I will just have a lie down for a while (Angela, 56 years, AS).

Box 1.7

I don't care what anyone says. I know that when I eat certain things like tomatoes or oranges my joints hurt more. When I've told the doctor she just smiles and I know what she's thinking but it happens every time. The same with the weather; I know what the day is like before I open the curtains in the morning (Claire, 59 years, RA).

The problem is that unless you have actually experienced living with FM it is hard for others to understand exactly what you are going through. When I meet others with FM, you don't have to explain it; they just know what you are going through (Kate, 54 years, FM).

Box 1.8

Even if I'm really tired I push myself to go out in the evening. I think living on my own I always try and plan into my day at least talking to someone or seeing someone, because otherwise I will go all day and I won't have talked with anyone (Claire, 29 years, AS).

I really do know what caused the problem. We had my daughter's wedding 3 weeks after I came out of hospital so you can imagine what I was doing. Things that I probably shouldn't have been attempting and going for longer period without resting to get things done. So I know I overdid things. I was absolutely shattered on the wedding day; I don't know how I got myself there, but I did and it was fantastic (Pam, 62 years, RA).

and exchanging experiences with other people living with rheumatic conditions leads to the development of shared community forms of truth and sense making (Box 1.7).

For healthcare professionals, understanding these community forms of truth can provide valuable insights into people's beliefs and understanding about a number of illness-related factors and can help occupational therapists to identify beliefs which may need to be addressed to increase the adoption of certain therapeutic interventions. As occupational therapists, we may seek to promote strategies such as pacing and energy conservation but, when located within the wider social context of people's lives, decisions to use such strategies are balanced against a host of competing demands and priorities. There are times when other things assume greater importance, and conscious decisions about a certain course of action are taken in full knowledge of the consequence (Box 1.8).

Situated learning does not necessarily mean not repeating mistakes or not doing things which make the condition worse but can enable a person to understand and prepare for the consequences of certain courses of action. A wide range of factors influence a person's decision to push themselves to their limits which include not wanting to let people down:

> I would rather leave everything and keep an appointment rather than phone up and say I can't make it. I have to be really ill and in an awful lot of pain. I would rather take double the pain killers and go and meet them, than say I'm not coming (Paul, 49 years, AS).

and the desire to continue to fulfil key roles and responsibilities:

> I feel it is my responsibility to try to do as many of the things now as I used to before I had RA, the personal things, the housework, cooking of the meals this sort of thing. Playing my part as a wife, mother and grandmother (Pam, 62 years, RA).

The narratives of people with rheumatic conditions often use terminology associated with combat such as 'fighting', 'battling' and 'not being defeated'. Independence is valued highly and asking for help is often associated with 'giving in'.

> If I'm honest I don't want to let my AS interfere with my life in any way. I want to just go on doing what I've always done and if I can't that would be like giving in. I think I see it as a bit of a challenge (Peter, 41 years, AS).

> I absolutely hate asking for help, it makes me feel like I am a burden on others. The other day I was watching my son do my garden and thinking about all the things he should be doing for his own family (George, 69 years, osteoarthritis).

The need to negotiate assistance within the family is not always an easy process. In the following extract, Karen, who is newly married, describes how she has recently employed a cleaner but has not told her husband:

> Well it's all done when he's at work. She comes here during the day and then any ironing I drop down during the day and she drops it off so he doesn't know at the moment (Kate, 34 years, RA).

This was due to the fact that she felt she should be fulfilling what she felt to be her duties as a wife and not wanting to 'let him down'. Clients may also have to confront the emotions associated with needing help from their children:

> I have this ongoing argument in my head that says, 'it's me that's got RA not the children'. I didn't have them to look after me (Brenda, 48 years, RA).

who, as Brenda went on to describe, can at times be both vocal and forthright in making their position clear:

> ...she's 14 and she said, 'well you know dad,' because she knew he was going to say something, 'well you know dad I've had a busy day and I don't know what Mum's done all day but I've been very busy,' Well you sort of curl up in a ball and laugh and cry at the same time (Brenda, 48 years, RA).

Thus it is that negotiating assistance is closely linked with saving face, the nuanced interplay of trying to fulfil desired occupational roles and thereby protecting valued occupational identities. People engage in complex and complicated calculations of how they balance what they have to do, what they can do and what they want to do. Being sensitive to the subtleties of these calculations is an important part of our therapeutic repertoire and is an essential part of facilitating occupational balance.

1.4   Summary

The focus of this book on lifestyle management highlights the fact that having a rheumatic condition is one facet of a person's life which can only be understood when located within the wider context of their personal narrative. The stories of people living with rheumatic conditions tell of struggles and challenges, but they also tell of achievements, of hopes and aspirations which have nothing to do with their impairment and of a desire to transcend the 'illness narrative' and to be understood as a person with many stories to tell. Successful occupational therapy management is predicated on understanding the multiple narratives a person has to tell and the influence that different facets of a person's life will have upon therapeutic interventions.

Resources

National Rheumatoid Arthritis Society

The National Rheumatoid Arthritis Society (NRAS) website contains a wide range of resources, including a section on personal narratives written by people living with RA describing the impact it has on their life. http://www.nras.org.uk/about_rheumatoid_arthritis/living_with_rheumatoid_arthritis/case_studies/female/default.aspx. Accessed on 14 November 2012.

Healthtalkonline

A specific section in healthtalkonline provides information about RA and people talking about their experience of living with and managing it. http://www.healthtalkonline.org/Bones_joints/Rheumatoid_Arthritis. Accessed on 14 November 2012.

References

Frank A (1995) *The Wounded Storyteller: Body, Illness and Ethics*. Chicago, IL: Chicago University Press.

Goldstein K, Kielhorner G, Paul-Ward A (2004) Occupational narratives and the therapeutic process. *Australian Journal of Occupational Therapists* 51:119–124.

Kleinman A (1988) *The Illness Narrative: Suffering, Healing and the Human Condition*. New York: Basic.

Mattingly C (1998) *Healing Dramas and Clinical Plots: The Narrative Structure of Experience*. Cambridge, UK: Cambridge University Press.

Chapter 2

Living with rheumatic diseases: the theoretical perspective

Margaret McArthur[1] and Lynne Goodacre[2]

[1]*University of East Anglia, Norfolk, United Kingdom;* [2]*Lancaster University Lancaster, United Kingdom*

2.1 Introduction

It is usual for healthcare professionals to draw on literature from the clinical health sciences to inform their practice; however, in this chapter, we aim to draw upon insights and perspectives into the experience of living with and managing a long-term condition (LTC) derived from the social sciences, specifically medical sociology.

Social processes play a central role in health and well-being, influencing, amongst other things, a person's beliefs about health and illness, their attitudes towards their body, their sense of self, and their life expectancy and opportunities. In a challenge to the domination of the biomedical model of illness, sociologists have offered an understanding of illness which is heavily influenced by interpretative approaches to research focusing on how a person, and their families and social networks, makes sense of an illness and how this process of sense making influences the actions they take (Nettleton 2006).

Client-centred occupational therapy practice informed by sociology of health and illness perspectives has the potential to contribute to therapists' understanding of people's experiences of living with and managing rheumatic conditions. In this chapter, we focus on the process of understanding what is happening and communicating that understanding to significant others, the impact of a rheumatic condition on a person's sense of self and insights into experiences of living and coping with an LTC.

2.2 Understanding and being understood

A strong thread running through sociological research associated with LTCs relates to how people make sense of what is happening to them in the early stages of disease

Rheumatology Practice in Occupational Therapy: Promoting Lifestyle Management, First Edition.
Edited by Lynne Goodacre and Margaret McArthur.
© 2013 John Wiley & Sons, Ltd. Published 2013 by John Wiley & Sons, Ltd.

onset. Closely associated to this is how, within the wider social context of partners, family, friends and colleagues, others also make sense of what is going on. The concepts of biographical disruption (Bury 1982; Bury 1991) and narrative reconstruction (Williams 1984, 1993) provide insights into these issues.

Biographical disruption

The work of Bury in the 1980s describing the onset of a chronic illness as a biographical disruption was seen as moving the sociology of illness from describing lay experiences of illness to theorising about them (Lawton 2003). Informed by research undertaken with people in the early stages of rheumatoid arthritis (RA), Bury (1982) described the onset of a chronic illness as a major disruptive event which leads a person to reappraise their biography, self-concept and life trajectory. He described how the often taken-for-granted assumptions a person makes about their body, their existence and aspects of their behaviour are challenged in a way which impacts not only on their 'structures of meaning' but also on relationships and resources.

To understand the context of the life trajectory, it is important for people to make meaning from their first experiences of having a medical condition which is potentially disabling and which, from a very early stage, has an effect on how they operate in their world. In this way, chronic illness is not an isolated aspect; more a continuing round of a never-ending story and is therefore an integrated aspect of the self. Howell (1998) suggests that meaning develops over time, has many influences and has a significant impact on the person's lived experience. The construction of meaning is influenced by a consideration of how the alteration or disappearances of valued elements of a person's identity has a profound effect on that identity. Complex skills are needed by the therapist and the client to understand meaning and the lived experience.

Within the context of biographical disruption, Bury highlighted the role of uncertainty in increasing the level of disruption which takes place especially with regard to the emergence and onset of a condition. As highlighted in Chapter 1, in many rheumatic conditions, uncertainty is a common experience and obtaining an actual diagnosis may take time due to the relapsing-remitting nature of early symptoms and confusion with other potential diagnosis. Bury and others (Ciambrone 2001; Lawton 2003; Pound et al. 1998) also emphasised the need to understand not only the meaning of an illness to the individual but also the context in which it occurs as the level of disruption experienced will vary from person to person depending upon their previous and current life experiences.

In later work, Bury made the distinction between meanings of *consequence*, the effects of an impairment on everyday life, and meanings of *significance*, the different connotations and imagery associated with an illness (Bury 1988). The emphasis on 'meaning' highlights the fact that diagnostic labels, outside of the clinical context, are imbued with culturally defined meanings and significance which impact not only on the individual concerned but also their families and wider social networks.

Whilst the concept of biographical disruption was seen as significant in terms of developing theory, its universal relevance has been challenged due to its focus on predominantly young people. The work of Sanders et al. (2002) suggested that the level of disruption people experience may relate to their location in the life course. Working with older people with osteoarthritis (OA), they suggested that symptoms of OA were perceived as a normal and integral part of participants' biographies rather than a major biographical disruption. This has subsequently been described by Williams as 'biographically anticipated' as opposed to biographically disruptive (Williams 2000).

Legitimation

Within the social science literature, the term 'legitimation' is used in a number of ways. Locker (1983) describes the process of legitimation as the process by which society acknowledges a person as having an impairment, i.e. their impairment and the challenges arising from it are accepted as credible and valid. It is common for people with rheumatic conditions to be challenged about the legitimacy of their impairment due to the lack of outwardly visible signs of illness coupled with the fact that they often do not comply with culturally held beliefs about 'arthritis' which is largely associated with older people. The other aspect of rheumatic conditions which can challenge their legitimacy is their variability; on some days, a person may be able to undertake activities independently whilst on other days they may require assistance. People with impairments like FM can also experience challenges about the legitimacy of their impairment due to negative social perceptions associated with conditions such as FM and chronic fatigue syndrome.

The legitimation of an impairment impacts upon a person's ability to mobilise the resources they may need to enable them to manage their impairment and their lives. Charmaz (1991) refers to those who watch a person becoming ill as audiences of interruption, i.e. those who are observing what is happening and making up their own minds about what they are observing, what kind of assistance to provide and how to respond. The kinds of resources referred to include things like the level of assistance and support received from work colleagues, assistance from the family and from statutory bodies to provide access to relevant services and benefits.

The concept of legitimation is utilised in a more focused way by Bury (1991), who uses the term to describe the process by which a person seeks to 'repair disruption and establish an acceptable and legitimate place for the condition' within their life. This is a more personal process of integrating illness into a personal biography in a way that gives it perspective and credibility.

A major factor influencing legitimacy is the receipt of a medical diagnosis which for many people confers legitimacy. Charmaz (1991, p. 24) uses the term 'diagnostic relief' to describe the experience of some people who have been given a diagnosis after a significant period of uncertainty. Living through an extended period of ill health lacking a diagnosis leaves a person vulnerable to not only the disbelief of others but also to self-doubt about whether their illness is real or imagined.

Narrative reconstruction

In 1984, Williams conducted a study on the basis of asking people with RA what they thought had caused their impairment. In the absence of a clear rationale provided by clinicians, Williams found that perceived causes were often located within the context of people's biographies. They were linked to past and current events in a way which provided, for the individual and those to whom they recounted their experience, a rational explanation about what was happening to them, a process of sense making described as narrative reconstruction. As healthcare professionals, insights into a person's narrative reconstruction can help to identify their beliefs about their impairment and inform approaches to therapeutic interventions.

When located within the social context of people's lives, there is a need to not only make personal sense of what is happening but also to convey this to others. People need to determine who they are going to tell and how much they are going to tell. Charmaz (1991) suggests that disclosure can be a strategic process designed to protect a person by maintaining a sense of control and power. This process can be observed in some people's unwillingness to tell employers or colleagues about their impairment for fear of the implications this may have on their job security or prospects for promotion.

Interruption, intrusion and immersion

The work of Kathy Charmaz has exerted a strong influence on understanding the experience of living with an LTC. In the early stages of impairment, Charmaz (1991) describes the experience of illness as comprising interruption, intrusion and immersion, emphasising that these do not necessarily occur in a linear sequence. Interruption refers to the onset of initial symptoms, the first sense of not being well which may or may not have an intrusive effect upon a person's life. The movement of symptoms from the background to the foreground of a person's life will usually prompt them to seek assistance with, at this stage in the illness trajectory, the hope of a full recovery.

Charmaz describes how the hope of recovery can be construed by healthcare professionals as denial when in fact it may be part of a person's journey to understanding the long-term nature of their impairment. The hope of recovery has implications for the timing of delivering self-management programmes as a person hoping for recovery will not be receptive to making lifestyle adjustments to accommodate an impairment which, in their minds, is short term. Developing an understanding of the long-term nature of illness has been described as mapping a new territory, 'The destination and map I had used to navigate before were no longer useful' (Frank 1995, p. 1). People are required to think differently about their body and their relationship with it, their future life plans and expectations.

The extent to which a person becomes immersed in their illness depends upon the intrusiveness of the symptoms they experience, treatment regimes and to some extent the person themselves. During periods of acute exacerbation, it is common for symptoms to become the focus of a person's life with gaining relief from relentless unremitting pain a priority; a person can become overwhelmed by and immersed in their pain. However, during periods of remission the level of intrusion reduces along with the level of immersion (Ulus et al. 2011). There are however some individuals who can become totally immersed in their illness which assumes a central part of their lives and their self-concept, they define themselves by their illness.

2.3   The impact of a rheumatic condition on a person's sense of self

An important factor for health professionals to consider is the effect of being in control on a person's self-concept. Self-concept is influenced through participation in, and is constituted by, the social world (Cohler 1982; Goffman 1963; Mead 1934; Polkinghorne 1988; Vallacher and Wenger 1987, 1989) so that we are what others have created. Taussig (1980) proposes that the physical manifestations of a disease signify more than the assessment of how well a body is functioning. He believes they also contribute to components of cultural and social relations, what Sacks (1991, p. xxix) meant when he talked about 'the junction of biology with biography'.

The presentation of self

People who acquire visible deformities later in life go through a process of re-identification influenced in part by the responses they experience within social contexts as a consequence of their appearance and self presentation (Goffman 1963). Prior to the onset of a rheumatic condition, people will have formed a perception about 'disabled people' and what it means to be disabled, which will range from positive to negative perceptions informed by personal and cultural perceptions (Swain et al. 2003). When a person acquires a disability, they then associate with their previously held beliefs as well as experience how others may respond to them differently:

> The most difficult thing was to be amongst my friends and see pitying, sympathetic looks. I hated it I really hated it. They were very kind and tried to be helpful but they overdid it. It felt like they didn't know how to approach me, people I'd been easy with for years didn't seem to know how to talk to me any longer.

Rather than being passive recipients of such experiences, Goffman (1963) described how people utilise a range of strategies to manage their appearance to minimise visible signs of disability and disfigurement. *Passing* is described as the 'management of undisclosed, discrediting information about the self' (Goffman 1968, p. 58) and is possible when there are no outwardly visible signs of disability; a person can choose whether or not to disclose information about themselves to others. Once there are visible signs of disability, people may develop skills in *covering* by which people attempt to prevent their disability from imposing upon social interactions, suggesting that the presentation of self can be likened to a performance (Goffman 1959). However, he acknowledges that it is possible for performers to be fully aware of the external identity defined by their performance and that this is not the full presentation of their self:

> I'm in a bar in [place name] with a bunch of people and a new person joins us and after a while says, 'What sort of person are you? Oh – very sensible shoes – I know'. I just keep thinking about it and it's made me kind of not want to go out.

Whilst Goffman's work has been highly influential in informing understanding of the management of identity, it has been criticised strongly by disability activists' writing due to its focus on how individuals seek to manage and minimise the impact of their disability as opposed to focusing at a societal level of challenging negative and discriminatory practices which lead people to feeling a need to hide their disability. Thomas describes the psychoemotional effects of disablism as socially imposed restrictions which shape personal identity and work along psychological and emotional pathways (Thomas 1999).

> I do feel self conscious, I see people looking at me because I walk funny, with my ankles but, I just put up with it. You've got to. People stare. I have people staring at my hands when I'm sat anywhere, this woman was looking at my hands and she looked at me and looked at my hands and then looked at me and I thought, 'you silly woman'. But I also thought 'oh god beam me up Scotty'.

Such encounters can have a negative psychological and emotional impact upon a person's identity, self-concept and confidence. When talking about his life in which he has accommodated childhood poliomyelitis, a car accident, subsequent carpal tunnel syndrome, arthritis and diabetes, Zola (1991, p. 2) explains that:

> I want at the very least to bring these personal bodily experiences closer to my center – not to claim that they constitute all of who I am, but that they are a central part of my identity; not that they explain all I have accomplished, but they are essential to understanding what I have done.

Like many people with disabilities, Zola does not want to deny that he has a disability but he does not want to be defined by that disability. He wants his achievements to be judged by who he is, not by what he has done *despite* his disability.

Investigating self-knowledge, or, more accurately, what clients think and know about themselves, helps in identifying the factors which inform the setting of goals and the exploration of whether specific forms of behaviour change are possible and desirable.

The contextual self

We do not live in or experience the same world as each other, but the worlds we inhabit and experience can be described and discussed. In fact, the differences are important to everyday understanding. The work of sociologists has provided important insights into how people with LTCs locate their experiences within the wider context of their lives, which includes the impact of age, class, gender, occupation, marital status and the type and extent of disability a person experiences (Charmaz 1991).

Sarup (1996, p. 38), when discussing the construction of identity, refers to Merleau-Ponty's proposal that a significant experience can lead to an identity based on that experience and that the experience can become a 'style of being'. This style of being and seeing and sensing significance can be regarded as an important way of defining context within an experience. It is in this way that past experiences and present circumstances determine the contextual construction of the definition of experiences.

When considering the context of health and significant experiences, Kleinman (1988, p. xiii) proposes that 'We can envision in chronic illness and its therapy a symbolic bridge that connects body, self and society'. The image of body, self and society can be interpreted as the contexts of health. The impact of a diagnosis is measured against the contexts of health that people develop from past experiences and present circumstances, and those experiences and the interpretation will be individual to each person.

The loss of self

Charmaz (1983) suggests that the sum total of the experience of having a chronic illness is often defined by physical suffering but highlights that people may also experience a loss of self. She describes self-concept as the organisation of attributes that have become consistent over time, proposing that the self is developed and maintained through social relations and socialisation. In this way, changes in self-concept occur throughout the life cycle. Charmaz proposes that people with LTCs can experience an erosion of their former self-image without necessarily experiencing the development of a new self-image due to reductions in social relationships and socialisation.

It is important to emphasise that whilst the concept of 'loss of self' is closely associated with the experience of living with chronic illness, the population from which Charmaz derived her early data were people who were severely disabled and/or housebound and therefore may not be representative of people who experience lower levels of activity limitation. However, some of the insights and perspectives are of relevance.

Charmaz also shows how living a restricted life and social isolation can focus attention on illness, highlighting the role of choice and freedom to pursue valued activities in reducing the experience of restriction. She identifies a number of factors which can pose restrictions upon a person's life, including the debilitating effects of treatment regimens, healthcare professionals not fully informing people of the choices open to them, disabling environmental barriers, discriminatory attitudes and practices, reduced income and variability and unpredictability of people's impairment.

Charmaz also discusses illness as an experience that shapes situations in which a person learns new definitions of self and often relinquishes old ones. A reduction in function can interfere with the public and private roles that have evolved to create that sense of self. It is within the philosophical underpinning of occupational therapy to consider the fulfilment of potential and achieving goals as these have personal meaning and all contribute to a person's self-image:

> I can't do the gardening anymore, I can't do any painting or anything like that … I do as much as I can and sometimes it's agony and sometimes it's frustrating … they're never done to my satisfaction anymore as they were when I was fit.

A loss of self-image and loss of ability to fulfil desired roles might result in an inability to define what is necessary to achieve autonomy. In addition, becoming disabled within desired roles may cause a loss of control.

> No one else notices it (dust) but it's irritating me. This is how I get moody I want things done, it's not just my house. They think the fairy does it! I guess it isn't really important but you can't tell my emotional system that because I still get worked up.

People with rheumatological conditions have many uncertainties surrounding the consequences of the disease (McArthur 2002). They can be thrust along a journey of *Self-discovery* and the impact of the things they find out about themselves, 'I didn't know I would feel like this'. This can force them to re-consider their *Self-definition* as they try to make meaning about their illness. This influences *Self-direction* with an impact on the decisions they make about what they can and can't do and what they do or don't want to do. With the potentially longstanding nature of rheumatological conditions, it is important to make every effort from the onset of the disease to help people to maintain a healthy self-image as this has a major impact on how they cope with the disease – if we cannot cure the disease, we have to help people to accommodate the consequences of the condition.

Even in the acute phase of a disease, people are already telling stories about an altered sense of self (McArthur 2002).

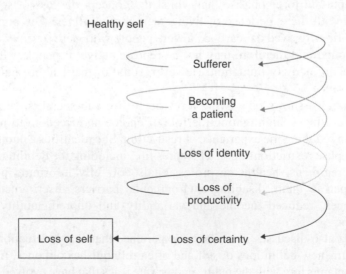

The story is as much about *being* as it is about *doing*.

The client embarks upon a journey in which they move from Healthy Self to Sufferer. Before they even seek treatment, people are playing a guessing and bargaining game.

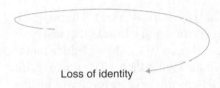

Healthy self

Sufferer

This is influenced by the healthcare system which facilitates the dynamic of Becoming a Patient including changes in routines and roles which places them in the sickness role.

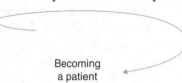

Becoming
a patient

The result is that clients can experience a loss of pre-morbid identity challenging their previously held and well-established ways of responding to life, feeling out of control.

Loss of identity

One important attack on identity is losing productive occupational roles with the accompanying reduction in the opportunity to practice skills they have, have social contact, a routine to follow, status and money.

Loss of
productivity

The compromise of valued roles results in a loss of certainty with a potential for a compromised self with a loss of familiar appraisal and coping strategies.

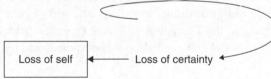

Loss of self   ◄   Loss of certainty ◄

Charmaz (1983) describes how clients draw upon past social experiences, cultural meanings and knowledge to engage in a mental dialogue about the meanings of their present physical and social existence.

> I've had an awful day today, can't concentrate and just want to be left alone. The reason is the fact that I have once again been drawn into the belief that I can live a normal live by going out everywhere that comes up, trips, theatre, going out with people. I can't. I have to live quietly and then I can cope, not too much activity all at once.

She proposes that the self-concerns become visible in chronic illness and that ill people become highly aware of previously taken-for-granted aspects of self because they have altered or disappeared, suggesting that through this mental dialogue a person's identity emerges through the experience of illness.

Helpless, hopeless, useless?

Some people with rheumatological conditions describe feelings of helplessness because they feel they have lost control over their lives, hopelessness through loss of choice and uselessness because they had lost options to demonstrate their perceived usefulness (McArthur 2002). The depth of feeling ranges from 'I strongly believe in positive thinking and concentrate on the things I can do. It's important to move on and try new things that otherwise you wouldn't have tried', to 'I live in quiet despair really…I want my old life back and I can't have that…'.

Being an expert, being a client: a balancing act

The expert client is an evolving concept (DoH 2001; Tattersall 2005). Thorne et al. (2000, p. 305) identify common health professional values and attitudes that can have an impact on living with and negotiating health care for an LTC. They identify that if health professionals undervalue client expertise in managing their LTC, it can result in 'mutual alienation in chronic illness care relationships'. Therefore, within this dynamic there is a fine balance between professional expertise and valuing the experience brought to the encounter by the client. Too much one way produces a submissive client reacting to expert opinion. Too much the other way creates a situation where the client is being asked to take too much responsibility for their illness.

Self-discovery and self-definition are often socially influenced. It is important to remember that it is difficult for both the client and the therapist to assess what is expected from the therapeutic encounter. Introspection by the client (and the therapist) may find a thoroughly conditioned self (Mead 1934) in that society as a whole has views about us that we unknowingly incorporate into our sense of self and our behaviours conform to those expectations. Clients will have developed an understanding of the role expected of someone who is, for example, ill/has arthritis/is off work, by the life events and health career they have had so far. Therapists will have an understanding of their role based on training, past personal and professional experiences and by interaction with role models.

A decision to change may reflect socially instilled values and preferences. Self-administered checks on the autonomy of the individual may themselves be products of socialisation. Reviews of these checks may also be socially tainted (Meyers 1989; Singelis and Brown 1995). If clients are expecting to be passive recipients of expert-led health care, then it will be a challenge for them to accommodate a therapeutic encounter where a partnership of care is suggested. Clients have a behavioural expectation developed on the basis of prior experience, or relatives' experiences of medical care. They generally expect the healthcare professionals to be in a position of power (Barry et al. 2001; Oliver 1996; Treichler et al. 1987). All of these factors combined with the quality of the available social support will influence the level of empowerment displayed by the client. A negotiated journey through service provision with a respect for the expertise that all bring to the encounter results in collaborative care (McArthur 2002).

2.4   The experience of living with a rheumatic condition

Moos (1984) identifies that people with a chronic illness commonly participate in a range of adaptive tasks, including the preservation of a satisfactory self-image, sense of achievement and/or competence and the retention of psychological equilibrium. This includes retaining control of negative feelings such as anxiety and anger, and fostering positive feelings such as hope and a sense of humour. These tasks are enhanced by the maintenance of positive meaningful relationships.

Thorne et al. (2000) discuss how chronic illness confronts people with major lifestyle adaptations which become the tool kit with which people react to and interact with their worlds. Much of the practice of occupational therapists working with people with rheumatic conditions relates to the development of skills and strategies, and therapists are often party to the numerous innovative ways in which people and their families overcome practical problems they may be experiencing.

In exploring how people respond to the challenges of living with LTCs, Bury highlighted the need for clarity in how the terms coping, strategy and style are used and made a clear distinction between them.

Definitions of coping, strategy and style (Bury 1991)

- Coping   The cognitive processes whereby the individual learns how to tolerate or put up with the effects of illness
- Strategy   The actions people take, or what people do in the face of illness, rather than the attitudes they develop
- Styke   The way people respond to, and present, important features of their illnesses or treatment regimens

Charmaz also provided detailed insights into the adjustments people make to accommodate an LTC as comprising *planning, tightening and modifying or organizing tasks and activities* (1991, p. 138) and describes how people make tradeoffs, reorder time and need to juggle and pace themselves.

Examples of making adjustments to accommodate an LTC can be seen in Table 2.1.

Many of the skills and adjustments derived from people's narratives about living with LTCs will be familiar to occupational therapists. Such narratives are also testament to the fact that whilst rheumatic conditions do have a major disruptive effect upon a person's life and their self-concept, many people maintain fulfilling lives in which they accommodate their impairment.

Mastery and occupational gain

Several studies have highlighted how, over time, people develop ways of managing and living with a rheumatic condition (Goodacre 2006; Shaul 1995; Stamm et al. 2009) and develop a level of mastery over it. Experience has taught them how to

Table 2.1   Making tradeoffs.

Simplifying tasks (which can involve a change in standards)	I let things go now that before would have had to be done and tell myself it doesn't really matter, I'm learning that a bit of dust doesn't kill anyone
Trading activities	If I'm going to choir in the evening I'll sit down for longer than my usual hour in the afternoon and I won't cook a big meal for the family in the evening, they sort themselves out that evening
	If we decide to go to the cinema or something, I do very little during the day so as to be able to go out at night and enjoy it
Staying at home	By the time I get in from work I just want to flop on the sofa. I'm pretty done in most days. I used to meet up with my mates once a week for a drink but it's ages since I've made it. All my energy is going into keeping my job at the moment
The tradeoffs that people make often impact upon partners, families and colleagues and may require organisation and also an increase in work for them	
Organisation of help	It comes down to being assertive I think, rather than sitting back and waiting for them to do it you shouldn't expect them to realise that you need help you need to say, 'can you help me with this please'. They can't read your mind can they?
Increasing work for others	We are like a well-oiled machine in the mornings each ofthe children have the things they need to do and Paul does quite a lot in the evenings as well
Reordering time	
In some instances, reordering time is possible	My boss has been really flexible and we have adjusted my hours so that I can come in for 9.30 instead of 8.30; that hour makes a massive difference in the morning. Then I have a shorter lunch break and we reduced my hours by a couple of hours per week
In some instance it isn't	My husband was working away and so I was reliant upon my son to help me get undressed. It was his night out with his mates so I sat and waited until gone eleven to go to bed. No matter how much I tried, I couldn't get my jumper over my head
Juggling and pacing	
	Do a bit and stop for a bit, do a bit and stop for a bit, that's how I get all my jobs done. If I work like that I'm ok but if I try to do everything in one go I've had it

overcome problems and manage their symptoms and also how to adjust their lifestyle and access the resources they require to maintain meaningful occupational roles.

Historically, the disease trajectory of a person with inflammatory arthritis has been characterised by progression of the impairment with associated increases in activity limitation. However, the introduction of anti-TNFα therapy has enabled many people with inflammatory arthritis to move from a trajectory of occupational loss to one of potential improvement. A number of studies exploring the experiences of people with RA and ankylosing spondylitis prescribed anti-TNFα medication have identified improvements in occupational performance and consequently an increased ability to fulfil important occupational roles within activities of daily living, leisure and productivity domains (McArthur et al. 2012; Stockdale and Goodacre 2009).

The introduction of anti-TNFα treatment is therefore a positive experience for most respondents. However, whilst there appears to be an assumption that becoming well is a trouble-free process, a number of challenges have been highlighted (McArthur et al. 2012) with which people require support, specifically with regard to defining appropriate goals and aspirations, managing ongoing symptoms and capitalising on reduced levels of activity limitations. People have to work hard to achieve mastery, and new levels of participation have to be established.

Occupational therapists enable people to accommodate and adapt to new occupational situations, but within current rheumatology practice, therapists may more usually be working with people experiencing occupational loss. The development of pharmaceutical interventions for inflammatory arthritis creates the need for therapists to review and revisit their therapeutic interventions. Understanding the narrative construction work which clients receiving anti-TNFα treatment undertake highlights the importance for moving away from a biomedical model of management for this group to one which seeks to support them in redefining their aspirations and developing the relevant skills and strategies to make a successful transition into increased levels of occupational engagement.

2.5 Acknowledge the loss, promote the gain

It is essential that occupational therapists remember that the influences on self are numerous and ongoing. Illness is experienced as a psychosocial process in which the inner dialogue changes and therefore the definitions of experience changes. The challenge confronting healthcare professionals is to protect against further loss through unrealised occupational potential, to promote a regained self and to develop strategies for partnership which involve a therapeutic alliance where the needs of all stakeholders (healthcare commissioners, service providers and service users) are understood. Quicker diagnosis can prevent people putting their coping strategies on hold whilst they hope they haven't got a rheumatological condition. Quicker access to new biologic therapies, where appropriate, can potentially reduce the functional impact of the inflammatory process.

Being open to people's stories will help us to listen to what is important to these people to ensure that realistic and understandable rehabilitation goals are agreed that are expressed in terms that have meaning for the person. Acknowledging the losses they have experienced and clearly understanding the performance demands of desired occupational roles will facilitate the re-establishment of these roles and so will also facilitate occupational gain. Setting the terms of the therapeutic encounter in this way will go some way to ensure that everyone understands what is expected of them.

In reviewing the contribution of medical sociologists to informing understanding of lay experiences of illness, Lawton concludes that they have emphasised the 'overlapping and interdependent nature of body, self and society, together with the importance of looking at timing, setting and individual biographies' (Lawton 2003, p. 36). This conclusion highlights the relevance of these perspectives to the client-centred holistic nature of occupational therapy practice and the role that sociological perspectives have played in informing our understanding of the personal experiences of living with and managing a rheumatic condition.

References

Barry CA, Stevenson FA, Britten N, et al. (2001) Giving voice to the lifeworld. More humane, more effective medical care? A qualitative study of doctor–patient communication in general practice. *Social Science & Medicine* 53(4):487–505.

Bury M (1982) Chronic illness as biographical disruption. *Sociology of Health and Illness* 4:167–182.

Bury M (1988) Meanings at risk: The experience of arthritis. In: Anderson R, Bury M (eds.) *Living with Chronic Illness: The Experiences of Patients and Their Families*. London: Unwin Hyman.

Bury M (1991) The sociology of chronic illness: A review of research and prospects. *Sociology of Health and Illness* 13:451–168.

Charmaz C (1983) Loss of self: A fundamental form of suffering in the chronically ill. *Sociology of Health and Illness* 5:168–195.

Charmaz C (1991) *Good Days Bad Days. The Self in Chronic Illness and Time*. New Brunswick, NJ: Rutgers University Press.

Ciambrone D (2001) Illness and other assaults on self: The relative impact of HIV/AIDs on women's lives. *Sociology of Health and Illness* 23:517–540.

Cohler BJ (1982) *Life Span Development and Behaviour*. New York: Academic Press.

Department of Health (DoH) (2001) *The Expert Patient. A New Approach to Chronic Disease Management for the 21st Century*. London: DoH. http://www.dh.gov.uk/en/Publicationsandstatistics/Publications/PublicationsPolicyAndGuidance/DH_4006801. Accessed on 11 November 2012.

Frank A (1995) *The Wounded Storyteller. Body, Illness and Ethics*. Chicago, IL: University of Chicago Press.

Goffman E (1959) *The Presentation of Self in Everyday Life*. New York: Doubleday.

Goffman E (1963) *Stigma: Notes on the Management of Spoiled Identity*. London: Penguin.

Goffman E (1968) *Stigma: Notes on the Management of Spoiled Identity*. Harmondsworth, UK: Pelican Books.

Goodacre L (2006) Women's perceptions of managing chronic arthritis. *British Journal of Occupational Therapy* 69(1):7–14.

Howell D (1998) Reaching to the depths of the soul: Understanding and exploring meaning in illness. *Canadian Oncology Nursing Journal* 8(2):12–16.

Kleinman A (1988) *The Illness Narrative: Suffering, Healing and the Human Condition*. New York: Basic Books.

Lawton J (2003) Lay experiences of health and illness: Past research and future agendas. *Sociology of Health and Illness* 25:23–40.

Locker D (1983) *Disability and Disadvantage. The Consequences of Chronic Illness.* New York: Tavistock Publications.

McArthur M (2002) *Unheard Stories, Unmet Needs: The Clinical and Educational Implications of Perceptions of Rheumatoid Arthritis.* Ph.D. thesis, Centre for Applied Research in Education, School of Education and Professional Development, University of East Anglia, Norfolk, UK.

McArthur M, Birt L, Goodacre L (2012) *An Investigation into the Experiences of Occupational Gain in People with Inflammatory Arthritis Receiving AntiTNFα Treatment.* London: United Kingdom Occupational Therapy Research Foundation, College of Occupational Therapists.

Mead GH (1934) *Mind, Self and Society: From the Standpoint of a Social Behaviourist.* Chicago, IL: University of Chicago Press.

Meyers DT (1989) *Self, Society and Personal Choice.* New York: Columbia University Press.

Moos RH (1984) *Coping with Physical Illness: New Perspectives.* New York: Plenum.

Nettleton S (2006) *Sociology of Health and Illness* (2nd edn.). Cambridge, UK: Polity Press.

Oliver MM (1996) *Understanding Disability: From Theory to Practice.* Basingstoke, UK: Macmillan.

Polkinghorne DE (1988) *Narrative Knowing and the Human Sciences.* Albany, NY: State University of New York Press.

Pound P, Gompertz P, Ebrahim S (1998) Illness in the context of older age: The case of stroke. *Sociology of Health and Illness* 20 489–506.

Sacks O (1991) *Awakenings.* London: Picador.

Sanders C, Donovan J, Dieppe P (2002) The significance and consequences of having painful and disabled joints in older age: Co-existing accounts of normal and disrupted biographies. *Sociology of Health and Illness* 2;227–253.

Sarup M (1996) *Identity, Culture and the Postmodern World* Edinburgh, UK: Edinburgh University Press.

Shaul MP (1995) From early twinges to mastery: The process of adjustment in living with rheumatoid arthritis. *Arthritis Care and Research* 8(4):290–297.

Singelis TM, Brown WJ (1995) Culture, self, and collectivist communication linking culture to individual behavior. *Human Communication Research* 21(3):354–389.

Stamm T, Lovelock L, Stew G, et al. (2009) I have a disease but I am not ill: A narrative study of occupational balance in people with rheumatoid arthritis. *Occupational Therapy Journal of Research:Occupation, Participation and Health* 29(1):32–39.

Stockdale J, Goodacre L (2009) 'It's magic stuff': The experiences of patients with ankylosing spondylitis taking anti-TNF-alpha medication. *Musculoskeletal Care* 7(3):162–177.

Swain J, French S, Cameron C (2003) *Controversial Issues in a Disabling Society.* Buckingham, UK: Open University Press.

Tattersall R (2005) The expert patient: A new approach to chronic disease management for the twenty-first century. *Clinical Medicine, Journal of the Royal College of Physicians* 2(3):227–229.

Taussig MT (1980) Reification and the consciousness of the patient. *Social Science Medicine* 14B:3–13.

Thomas C (1999) *Female Forms.* Buckingham, UK: Open University Press.

Thorne SE, Nyhlin KT, Paterson BL (2000) Attitudes toward patient expertise in chronic illness. *International Journal of Nursing Studies* 37(4):303–311.

Treichler PA, Frankel RM, Kramarae C, et al. (1987) Problems and problems: Power relationships in a medical encounter. In: Mayor BM, Pugh AK (eds.) *Language, Communication and Education.* London: Croom Helm in Association with the Open University.

Ulus Y, Akyol Y, Tander B, et al. (2011) Sleep quality in fibromyalgia and rheumatoid arthritis: Associations with pain, fatigue, depression, and disease activity. *Clinical Experiments in Rheumatology* 29(6 Suppl 69):S92–S96.

Vallacher RR, Wegner DM (1987) What do people think they're doing? Action identification and human behaviour. *Psychological Review* 94(1):3–15.

Vallacher RR, Wegner DM (1989) Levels of personal agency: Individual variation in action identification. *Journal of Personality and Social Psychology* 57(4):660–671.

Williams G (1984) The genesis of chronic illness: Narrative reconstruction. *Sociology of Health and Illness* 6(2):175–200.

Williams G (1993) Chronic illness and the pursuit of virtue in everyday life. In: Radley A (ed.) *Worlds of Illness. Biographical and Cultural Perspectives on Health and Disease*. London: Routledge.

Williams S (2000) Chronic illness as biographical disruption or biographical disruption as chronic illness? Reflections on a core concept. *Sociology of Health and Illness* 22:40–67.

Zola IK (1991) Bringing our bodies and ourselves back in. Reflections on a past, present, and future 'Medical Sociology'. *Journal of Health and Social Behaviour* 32(3):1–16.

Chapter 3

Understanding rheumatic diseases: the occupational therapy perspective

Margaret McArthur

School of Allied Health Professions, University of East Anglia, Norfolk, United Kingdom

3.1   The centrality of occupation

As an occupational therapist, my professional practice has been based on the belief that everyday occupations may be used to prevent or accommodate disability as occupations are required to support participation in desired roles.

> *Occupation* – 'specific chunks of activity within the ongoing stream of human behaviour' (Yerxa et al. 1990, p. 5)

Wilcock (1995) suggests that such activities are culturally sanctioned, primary organisers of time and resources, and involvement in activity enables individuals to control and adapt to their occupational identities. They include everything from getting up in the morning, to playing the flute, to doing 'nothing'. These purposeful activities can be synthesised as doing, being, becoming (Hammell 1998) and belonging (Rebeiro et al. 2001).

> *Doing* – engagement in purposeful and meaningful activity (Hammell 2004)
> *Being* – the meaning, value and intentionality ascribed to activity, a 'rediscovery of oneself' (Wilcock 1999)
> *Becoming* – the aspiration of who or what someone would wish to become over time (Hammell 2004)
> *Belonging* – the contribution of social interaction, support and the sense of being included to occupational performance (Rebeiro et al. 2001)

Rheumatology Practice in Occupational Therapy: Promoting Lifestyle Management, First Edition.
Edited by Lynne Goodacre and Margaret McArthur.
© 2013 John Wiley & Sons, Ltd. Published 2013 by John Wiley & Sons, Ltd.

The common factor is that occupation is a purposeful use of time. It uses energy and engages interest and attention. It can encompass many aspects including work, leisure, family, cultural, self-care and rest activities.

3.2   Occupational potential

Difficulties with performing desired activities have an impact on health and well-being (Parnell and Wilding 2010). Therefore, a person's assessment of the likelihood that they will be able to fulfil their desired occupational potential can be the starting point of most occupational therapy encounters.

> *Occupational potential* – 'future capability, to engage in occupation towards needs, goals and dreams' (Wilcock 1998, p. 256)

Occupations and roles are entwined and people adopt and perfect their occupations to support their occupational roles. So, for example, when one client talks about going swimming, she describes it as an activity she could share with her family, as a useful way to fill her time, and as a replacement for the therapy she feels she needs to ameliorate the biomechanical consequences of having a rheumatological condition. When another client talks about sport, he acknowledges that there is the benefit of physical exercise to offset the impact of his arthritis, but equally as important to him was the opportunity for him to try to win, describing himself as a very competitive man.

3.3   Occupational science

One way of ensuring that client need is more fully addressed is by working within a framework informed by occupational science.

> *Occupational science* – the study of the human need to be occupied (Christiansen 1994)

Occupational science has come to the fore in the last two decades. Evidence suggests that occupational therapists have been striving to work within this theoretical framework in general (Christiansen 1999; Haley and McKay 2004; Keilhofner 2002; Wagman et al. 2012; Wilcock 1998; Yerxa et al. 1990) and whilst working with people with rheumatological conditions in particular (Alsaker and Josephsson 2003; Forhan and Backman 2010; Stamm et al. 2004, 2009).

What the research discusses is the *extent* to which occupational science needs to be operationalised in the work of occupational therapists.

Occupational science assumes that people have a *capacity* to perform daily occupational roles and a *need* to perform those roles (Ilott 1995).

Occupational form – 'the pre-existing structure that elicits, guides, or structures human performance' (Nelson 1987).
Occupational performance – an observable action or behaviour (Nelson 1987)

The challenge is understanding what prevents or enhances occupational performance and how social, cultural and political structures affect those valued occupations (Kepnen and Kielhofner 2006).

3.4   Understanding need

If occupational science is a study of what people do, occupational therapy is about helping people to do those things that are important to them. Any disease can potentially have an effect on what people are able to do. Therefore, within the therapeutic intervention, it is essential to find out what clients want to do. In chronic illness, making sense and meaning may be especially difficult, as the illness may be so preoccupying that it dominates the usual ways of constructing meaning. Clients *doing* really matters, but *what* they do is not as important as 'the acknowledgement that occupation is pregnant with meaning' (Clark et al. 1991, p. 301). Therefore, everyday occupations are important not only for their practical role but also because they contain accumulated meanings and the importance of continuing to engage in activities that matter. Therefore, occupational therapists need to understand the influences that shape the way that clients interpret themselves within their view of the world (Mattingley 1991), thereby honouring 'the power of ordinary experiences within the context of health care' (Clark et al. 1991, p. 300). People will benefit from a more equal sharing of the definition of meaning to enable them to have space to fully establish what they need to understand, in order to cope with their condition.

People with rheumatic conditions experience challenges in a range of activities (NICE 2009) in domains of activities of daily living (ADL) (Katz 1995; Linden and Bjorklund 2010; Van Vollenhoven et al. 2010), productivity (Backman 2004; Bansback et al. 2012; Gobelet et al. 2007; Keat et al. 2008; Verstappen et al. 2010; Yelin et al. 2003) and leisure activities (Da Costa et al. 2003; Ozgul et al. 2006; Reinseth et al. 2011). In particular, they experience challenges to occupational engagement and are less likely to engage in active work and leisure activities and are more likely to spend a larger proportion of their time in ADL, passive leisure and at rest (MacKinnon et al. 1994).

Action identification

Occupational therapists consider the *person* in the *situation* where what they do and what they say are ways of *knowing* and *being*. Any action can be represented (identified) in a variety of ways. Making the bed in the morning can mean: the start of the day; evidence of good house care skills; a need to maintain order and control; or an irritation because someone else should have done it. For someone with a rheumatic condition who has morning stiffness, it could mean any of those things, but if the task cannot be completed it could also mean: another thing they can't do; a need to get up earlier in the morning to achieve it because things take longer to do; another symbol of how their family does not support them or a confirmation of the positive regard of a significant other because they do it without being asked.

Action identification (AI) theory (Vallacher and Wegner 1987, 1989) proposes that people will concentrate on one main reason for what they are doing, such as 'start of the day' – the *prepotent identity*. It is the identity that comes most easily to the person when asked 'What are you doing?' There are *low-level* identities, which indicate *how* a task is done (e.g. hospital corners), and *high-level* identities, which are based on a more general understanding of the task (good house care skills) which signify *why* the task is done. Occupational therapists are under pressure to address the 'how' in an effort to, say, discharge a client from hospital or keep them in the community whilst they also want to attend to the 'why' to ensure that the occupational role needs are being met.

The second AI principle is that people consider their high-level identity when looking for *meaning* for their actions. However, when a person cannot do what they want to do, they tend to view the task as its component parts and so go back to the 'how' rather than the 'why'. The low-level identities are in fact an essential element as people gain a sense of themselves by being able to *do* things. 'Being' and 'doing', even at this level, are closely intertwined.

This process of identifying actions is familiar to occupational therapists used to breaking tasks down into component parts. This activity analysis enables the therapist and the client to plan a therapeutic programme within the reach of the client's present occupational performance. The aim is to consolidate and rehabilitate that performance. One of the problems is that people do not always identify their action until after it has happened, or once the action is complete they place a different interpretation upon it (Vallacher and Wegner 1987). This will be a complication when trying to set an agenda with a client. This could be addressed by therapists being aware of it whilst listening to their clients' stories, using the reformulation and reiteration inherent in the stories as a way of facilitating identification of goals.

AI proposes that a person can move from high-level to low-level and low-level to high-level identities. However, it is very difficult to move from high-level to high-level identities, that is, once a person has decided why they do something it is difficult to change that perception. To achieve a change in high-level identification, it is necessary to work at the low-level stage. For example, if someone with a rheumatic condition assumes a high-level identity of *I cannot take control of my disease*, it can be broken down into the various aspects of being out of control (Figure 3.1).

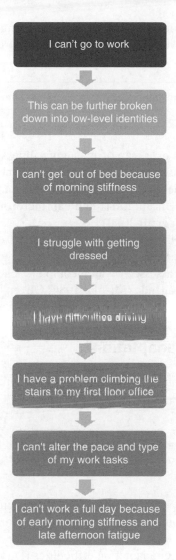

Figure 3.1 Example of action identification.

If occupational therapists are able to address any one of these elements and some return to work is effected, then the client's perception of 'not being in control of the disease' will be altered. There is then a possibility that regaining of control can be reviewed and transferred to other elements of life.

3.5 Occupational identity

Improvements in occupational performance are best achieved when occupation-based activities are used (Landa-Gonzalez and Molnar 2012) because developing identity through occupations are 'not just key to being a person, but to being a *particular* person' and those identities help to create meaningful lives (Christiansen 1999).

> *Occupational identity* – 'who one is and wishes to become as an occupational being' (Keilhofner 2002)

Thus it is that identity acts as a way of managing illness experiences (Alsaker and Josephsson 2003). So, for example, change in or retirement from productivity roles can impair occupational identity, but that impairment can be compensated for with desired leisure activities (Unruh 2004) and can therefore be a significant way of coping with illness (Unruh et al. 2000).

Therefore, occupational therapists assess what clients can or cannot do *but* often within the confines of an available service. It has been suggested that such confines can result in client needs being assessed by an incomplete 'checklist' rather than through their own (more complete) agenda (Mishler 1984; Oliver 1996; Treichler et al. 1987) even with the emerging policy initiatives on client-centred services (Chapter 4).

3.6   Occupational adaptation

The review, re-establishment or re-configuration of identity is facilitated by occupational adaptation.

> *Occupational adaptation* – the development of competence in occupational functioning, most pronounced in periods of transition (Schkade and Schulz 1992).

Adaptation can be strongly influenced by how the rheumatic condition developed: a steady development of symptoms without significant remission seems to facilitate a less challenging and gradual adaptation whilst acute onset with remission and relapse pattern creates greater adaptation difficulties (Dubouloz et al. 2008; Schkade and Schulz 1992). The process of adaptation is also influenced by factors such as the efficacy of medication, age, support of others and the meanings ascribed to suggested interventions, for example, the need to pace and rest conflicting with a personal schema of 'getting the job done' or the use of assistive devices being seen as a loss of independence (Dubouloz et al. 2008).

3.7   Occupational balance

Part of the process of adaptation is the assessment and facilitation of occupational balance. Occupational balance and its accompanying involvement of physical, psychological and social aspects of a person's engagement with the world is an important factor in maintaining health (Christiansen and Matuska 2006; Stamm et al. 2009; Wagman et al. 2012).

> *Occupational balance* – a balance of what HAS to be done against the things that people would LIKE (Stamm et al. 2004)

Stamm et al. (2004) found that people viewed occupational balance in different ways, with some seeing the success in achieving occupational balance despite their arthritis as a positive experience whilst those who felt that their arthritis controlled them had a negative view of occupational balance. Persson et al. (2011), when researching pain behaviours, identified that people gave up an occupation when symptoms increased unless the occupation was so important that the symptom was accepted or ignored.

3.8   Occupational gain

Occupational gain is important as it can help to redress that balance.

> *Occupational gain* – the improvement in functional, psychological and social ability to participate in activities.

Occupational gain for people with rheumatic conditions is about re-establishing previously valued occupational performance elements to enable people to fulfil important occupational roles (and therefore identity) or being able to engage in new occupations (McArthur et al. 2012). So, Jane, following a positive response to anti-TNFα medication, explains that she can '…take the children out for a day to a theme park', which has an impact on her occupational role, 'before I just used to be the bag person, I looked after the bags', and this has reaffirmed her occupational identity '…it's like being a teenager all over again'.

Occupational gain can be against a long-term trajectory of possible occupational deprivation. However, gain does not necessarily mean the return to pre-morbid function but can be about doing things that matter in whatever way they can be done (Knittle et al. 2011). Therefore, we need to be alert to the self-assessment of whether there is satisfactory occupational gain to underpin identity, especially as what might be acceptable to one person may be unacceptable to others (Hewlett 2003). In addition, occupational gain is heavily influenced by the chance to take supported risks (against a background of people with rheumatic conditions being risk-averse), influenced by choice and control and geared towards the development or maintenance of skills whilst fulfilling cultural norms. These performance modification demands are a central challenge to clients (Dubouloz et al. 2008) and need to be underpinned by the correct level of information delivered at the right time (Stamm et al. 2004).

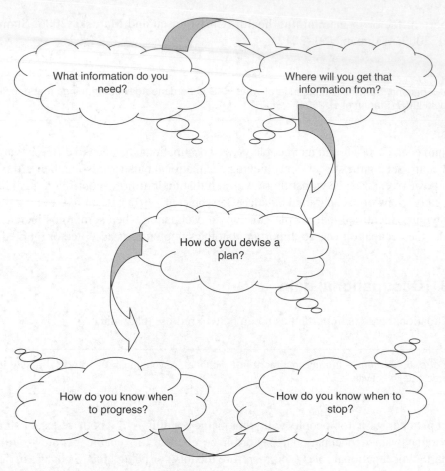

Figure 3.2   Clinical reasoning decision-making process.

3.9   Clinical reasoning – the thinking that guides practice

Clinical reasoning is the foundation of effective professional practice and where reasoning is absent interventions enter the 'realm of guesswork and become habit (at best) and fancy (at worst)' (Stephenson 2012, p. 76). Keeping up to date with current evidence has an essential part to play in the current developing commitment to continuing professional development which facilitates the development of clinical reasoning (McArthur and Mason 2012).

This reasoning is an integration of a wide variety of information sources such as client narrative, standardised and non-standardised assessment, research evidence, clinical audit, policy directives, input from other health professionals and feedback from family members. It is informed by instinct, comparison with past experiences, reflection-in-action and reflection-on-action. Even with all these information sources, it is vital that we can clearly articulate our decision-making to key stakeholders such as clients, other health professionals and commissioners of our services.

Whenever we meet a client, we are going through a number of decision-making processes to inform our understanding of their individual circumstances (Figure 3.2). A number of factors influence clinical reasoning (Schell 1998):

- *Diagnostic* – How do I/they know what it is?
- *Predictive* – How much better/worse can they become?
- *Procedural* – How will I go about 'treating' it?
- *Pragmatic* – What resources do I have?
- *Narrative and Prioritising* – What do they want to do…and in what order?
- *Conditional* – What are the physical/social/psychological contexts?
- *Ethical* – How do I choose morally defensible action given competing interests and so weigh up the benefits and risks to client, to other clients and to health to services in general? (Box 3.1)

When considering what to do with a client, a number of questions should always be posed:

1 What are the person's occupational performance concerns?
2 What is the person's occupational performance status and potential?
3 What can be done to improve occupational performance?

The clinical reasoning which could inform those questions is shown in Figure 3.3.

Box 3.1 Clinical reasoning case study

Sue is 42 years old. She has been referred from the rheumatology clinic for splinting. She works part time as a garden consultant in a local garden centre. She spends any free time engaged in gardening activities and regularly attends the local gardening club, and tries to attend a number of national flower shows each year.

She is concerned that when she is outside she develops a rash on her face. Also she complains that in cold weather her hands 'seize up', and this prevents her from gardening. In the last 3 months, her neck and shoulders ache and feel stiff. She has had a corresponding proximal muscle weakness, and this is worst in the morning. By the middle of the afternoon, she has generalised myalgia and arthralgia. Sue has experienced some chest pain and was worried that she was having a heart attack. She is also concerned that she seems to be losing patches of hair on her head.

Sue has noticed that her right arm has painfully restricted movement, for example, in the morning she can't reach to get the cereal box off a kitchen shelf above shoulder height without shoulder pain which radiates to the elbow. Turning her neck to reverse the car in the morning is restricted, with some right-sided pain, which spreads to the upper trapezius region. She is right-hand dominant.

For the last month, she has been experiencing a general feeling of malaise with fatigue, anorexia and feeling low in mood. She is noticeably upset when she attends the department. She doesn't think that her GP believes her when she describes her symptoms. Sue feels that her family are losing patience with her because she is sometimes too tired to join in family activities.

She has been reasonably healthy apart from a number of miscarriages in the past.

CLINICAL REASONING	
Clinical reasoning and occupational performance focus:	
1. What are the person's occupational performance concerns?	
2. What is the person's occupational performance status and potential?	
3. What can be done to improve occupational performance?	
Diagnostic	Diagnosed with systemic lupus erythematosus (SLE) 11 months after onset of symptoms by: complete blood count (CBC), antinuclear antibody panel (ANA), pattern of joint involvement, mild erosive changes on X-ray, presence of pain and fatigue, photosensitivity, hair loss and past miscarriages.
Predictive (2)	Good prognosis that has improved markedly over the last 20 years because of improvements in treatment. Treatment early in the course of the illness improves long-term progress. About 85–95% of people with SLE survive 10 years, and many people have a normal life span. SLE that develops laterin life is generally less serious than SLE that strikes in childhood or young adulthood (Bertsias et al. 2008). Prognosis would be reviewed if Sue developed haemolytic anaemia, heart, lung, kidney or central nervous system involvement.
Pragmatic (2,3)	Taking into account local, national and policy drivers (Chapter 4).
Prioritising (1,2)	Establishing what needs to be done first. Sue wants to stay in work to deal with work issues as a priority; challenges to family roles are an equal priority.
Narrative (1,2,3)	Sue is very worried that she will have to give up gardening which is a valued activity. She is also frightened, furious, guilty, ashamed of not being able to fulfil employee, wife, parent and friend roles. Greenberg et al. (1999) considered how compromises to the social self produce feelings of guilt. They suggested that protecting self-esteem can reduce anxiety and so reduce physiological arousal in response to subsequent threats. Family and friends – frightened, angry, ashamed of their impatience. Therapist – what are the performance elements that are essential to allow Sue to do what she wants/needs to do? Have I seen a case like this before?
Conditional (1, 2, 3)	Tiring job. Need to assess how much control Sue has over the pace and type of activities required for the job. Fearful employers – take into account the Equality Act 2010 when discussing reasonable adjustments (Chapter 13). Health professionals – SLE has a reputation for being both mysterious and serious despite the fact that many people with SLE have relatively mild disease. It is a striking feature of SLE that the severity of joint pain may be out of proportion to what there is to find on examination. This feature may sometimes lead to the client being doubted about the veracity of their symptoms. Relationship with husband and family – Fatigue is a common presentation and can be very disruptive to family relationships.
Procedural (1, 2, 3)	Assessment (Chapter 5) Education for Sue, family and employer about condition Splinting? Review the evidence base (Chapter 12) Pain and fatigue management (Chapters 7, 8, 9, 10, 11 and 12) Joint protection (Chapters 7 and 8) Vocational assessment and possibly vocational rehabilitation (Chapter 11) Sunscreen, wearing a hat and other strategies to overcome photo-sensitivity
Ethical (3)	Inability to engage in meaningful occupations will have significant health consequences so inadequate treatment has an important ethical dimension

Figure 3.3   Clinical reasoning worked example.

3.10   Personal perspectives

Therapists can have differing views and priorities depending on their stage of development and their work focus (Gibson et al. 2000). To explore this, the final part of this chapter presents personal perspectives of an occupational therapy student, a specialist rheumatology occupational therapist and an occupational therapy researcher.

Student occupational therapist

Preparing for the rheumatology role – As a third year occupational therapy student eagerly awaiting the latest placement allocations, I was delighted to find out I was off to the rheumatology department of a local acute hospital. I was apprehensive as to whether I would be able to make the smooth transition to third year student standards and whether what I had learned from previous placement experiences would transfer to this role. A pre-placement visit and pre-reading allayed my fears.

Moving from novice to practitioner – My observations over the first few days raised further questions within myself about the confidence clients may have in my abilities as a student occupational therapist and whether I would be able to overcome this potential barrier, especially as they were the experts in their condition and I was a novice. It was important for me to try to alleviate these concerns by being honest regarding my limitations and reassuring the clients that further support and advice was readily available through my practice educator if required. In reality, I found that by appearing confident and communicating directly and honestly I was able to develop an effective relationship with the clients.

Occupation-focussed therapy – When working with people who have long-term rheumatological conditions, I became acutely aware of the impact these can have on their life including physical well-being, home life, relationships, work, leisure and self-care. This enabled me to further develop knowledge and clinical skills, including assessment, goal setting, grading activities, the use of occupational therapy models and splinting. This field particularly offered me the opportunity of working in a truly holistic manner, something I have not always found in other clinical areas. This approach opened up my eyes to the difference occupational therapy can make, with our philosophy of seeing clients as people rather than focusing on the label of a condition. The true value of our profession really comes to the fore in this area as we are able to work side-by-side with people to jointly identify what is important to them in their lives and finding ways around enabling their occupational performance.

I found rheumatology occupational therapy extremely rewarding, and it was a real turning point in my progression towards becoming a newly qualified practitioner. I was able to confirm to myself the purpose and value of my chosen profession by seeing tangible evidence of the impact facilitating occupational performance can have on a person's well-being. I found I was able to draw on experiences from previous placements such as effective communication, information gathering, problem-solving and working with other members of the team. I was able to build on this with practice, which meant I finished this placement with increased confidence in my own abilities and looking forward to my future career as an occupational therapist.

Specialist rheumatology occupational therapist

Working as a clinical and professional lead for rheumatology services in a non-acute NHS hospital I find that 60–70% of my time is clinical, with the remainder focusing on management, service development, audit and research.

Change in approach – Over the past decade, there have been significant changes in my role. Routine inpatient rehabilitation for people with a newly diagnosis of a rheumatic condition is rare due to better medical management and the transition to community-based care. Delivery of core interventions such as self-management techniques and splinting is changing to embrace group work, goal setting and motivational interviewing techniques. The focus of occupational therapy has always been on self-care with the client becoming the expert although its importance is only just being acknowledged in the wider policy arena.

Is better good enough? – Anti-TNFα medication heralded more effective disease control and the possibility that fewer newly diagnosed clients develop chronic musculoskeletal changes that irrevocably impair function and quality of life. Whilst clients are certainly better, I wonder whether they are achieving their maximum occupational potential, so our intervention is vital to help them optimise on improved pharmaceutical control and assist those at the more severe end of the disease spectrum who cannot benefit from these medications.

Commissioning and evidence-based practice – I work within a broad scope of practice. Whilst this confers a great deal of professional freedom, it can make it more difficult to define my role. I am concerned that we are at risk of core interventions being adopted by other health professionals without the benefit of the full occupational performance focus. This is compounded by the changes in commissioning of services. There is a growing reliance on quality research and particularly randomised-controlled trials (RCTs) to justify the commissioning of services. Rheumatology occupational therapy has a lack of quality evidence to support current interventions. Splinting and hand exercises, two of our core practice areas, are not well evidenced and continue to be hotly debated. This has led to restricted development of evidence-based practice (EBP) and placed services with little or poor quality evidence at risk of being de-commissioned. We also need to consider how we can further develop our role, for example, exclusion from supplementary and independent prescribing legislation has prevented occupational therapists from engaging in emerging practitioner roles. On the plus side, my workload has seen a significant increase in diagnosis of hypermobility syndrome, fibromyalgia and other non-specific chronic pain conditions. None of these respond well to pharmaceutical management alone, so they will all continue to need occupational therapy, commonly as part of a multidisciplinary team approach, to maximise self-management and quality of life.

Occupational therapists have the knowledge and skills to make a vital contribution to rheumatology health services. To secure the future of occupational therapy as a core part of rheumatology services, we need to work in collaboration with other allied health professionals and researchers at operational, national and strategic levels to ensure that EBP is implemented and occupational therapy services continue to be commissioned.

Occupational therapy researcher

My experiences of rheumatology research are against a background of the challenges of gaining funding from a research culture that still tends to favour the RCT as the gold standard within an ever-changing health and social care environment that faces the demands of providing a top-notch service where more needs to be delivered with reduced resources.

What should we be doing? – My research manifesto is to meet the clients', therapists', commissioners' and policy makers' needs and to continue to promote mixed methods research that considers both efficacy and the experience of interventions. I am not denying the importance of producing cost-effective interventions with measurable effects, but there needs to be a continuing development of a more nuanced view because if insufficient attention is paid to the experiences of the people involved in the intervention it will seriously affect the efficacy of that intervention. My aim is always to present issues that would be stimulating and provide explanations that made good sense.

How should we be doing it? – Equally as important I want to ensure that rheumatology occupational therapy continues to develop its evidence base to underpin practice. We should not be backward in coming forward with the confidence that we have excellent research skills and important research questions to ask, which will not only benefit our practice but will influence health and social care policy and practice. We are developing a rich and robust research culture, and occupational therapist researchers have an increasing role to play at all levels from supporting pre-registration students to become more and more immersed in EBP, to postgraduate opportunities such as clinicians being involved in research partnerships and engaging in MSc level study and then on to an increasing number of occupational therapists being awarded PhDs. We have moved from being collaborators on other people's research projects to being grant holders in our own right and on to leading programmes of research, attracting funding from major funding bodies. There is an ever-increasing expectation for our research to be disseminated widely by publication, conference, stakeholder and public engagement activities.

To infinity and beyond – All these levels of research are important building blocks for our professional research identity so that we are not only responding to current research agendas but are also helping to shape emerging agendas of the future. I find the possibilities exciting, scary and exhausting in equal proportions as it is a responsibility to funders, our colleagues, our professional identity and of course our clients, but with a fair wind behind me I am up for the challenge.

So, in conclusion, to work within a client-centred and occupational focus, we need to not only assess a person's capacity to perform occupational roles but also to look very closely at a person's need to perform those roles. It would follow that with their core skills of activity analysis, occupational therapists are able to help clients to ascertain which activities are desirable for their maximal well-being and what adaptation (physical, psychological, environmental) needs to take place to allow those activities to be continued. In doing so, they take full account of the fact that performance of key occupational roles is partly influenced by a range of important factors. However, the resulting behaviour is also affected by, and has an effect on, the tasks to be performed and the environment within which the occupational performance takes place. It is the task of the therapist, therefore, to foster successful occupational behaviour to develop clients' motor abilities, self-concepts and social identities and help them re-define their sense of self and so open up new possibilities for the future (Kielhofner and Forsyth 1997).

Resources

COT Hot Topics. http://www.cot.co.uk/hot-topics/hot-topics. Accessed 19 November 2012.
Higgs J, Jones M (2000) *Clinical Reasoning in the Health Professions* (2nd edn.). Oxford: Butterworth Heinemann.
Mattingley C, Fleming MN (1994) *Clinical Reasoning. Forms of Inquiry in Therapeutic Practice.* Philadelphia, PA: FA Davis Co.
Molineux M (ed.) (2004) *Occupation for Occupational Therapists.* Oxford: Blackwell.

References

Alsaker S, Josephsson S (2003) Negotiating occupational identities while living with chronic rheumatic disease. *Scandinavian Journal of Occupational Therapy* 10:167–176.
Backman C (2004) Employment and work disability in rheumatoid arthritis. *Current Opinion Rheumatology* 16:148–152.
Bansback N, Zhang W, Walsh D, et al. (2012) Factors associated with absenteeism, presenteeism and activity impairment in patients in the first years of RA. *Rheumatology* 51:375–384.
Bertsias G, Ioannidis JP, Boletis J, et al. (2008) EULAR recommendations for the management of systemic lupus erythematosus. *Annals of Rheumatic Diseases* 67(2):195–205.
Christiansen C (1994) Classification and study in occupation. A review and discussion of taxonomies. *Journal of Occupational Science: Australia* 1(3):3–21.
Christiansen CH (1999) The Eleanor Clarke Slagle Lecture: Defining lives: Occupation as identity: An essay on competence, coherence and the creation of meaning. *American Journal of Occupational Therapy* 53:547–558.
Christiansen CH, Matuska KM (2006) Lifestyle balance: A review of concepts and research. *Journal of Occupational Science* 13:49–61.
Clark FA, Parham D, Carlson ME, et al. (1991) Occupational science: Academic innovation in the service of occupational therapy's future. *American Journal of Occupational Therapy* 45(4):300–310.
Da Costa D, Lowensteyn I, Drista M (2003) Leisure-time physical activity patterns and relationship to generalized distress among Canadians with arthritis or rheumatism. *Journal of Rheumatology* 30:246–284.

Dubouloz CJ, Vallerand J, Laporte D, et al. (2008) Occupational performance modification and personal change among clients receiving rehabilitation services for rheumatoid arthritis. *Australian Occupational Therapy Journal* 55:30–38.

Forhan M, Backman C (2010) Exploring occupational balance in adults with rheumatoid arthritis. *OTJR: Occupation, Participation and Health* 30(3):133–141.

Gibson D, Velede B, Hoff T, et al. (2000) Clinical reasoning of a novice versus an experienced occupational therapist: A qualitative study. *Occupational Therapy in Health Care* 12(4):15–31.

Gobelet C, Luthi F, Al-Khodairy AT, et al. (2007) Work in inflammatory and degenerative joint diseases. *Disability and Rehabilitation* 29(17):1331–1339.

Greenberg J, Solomon S, Pyszcynski T, et al. (1999) Why do people need self-esteem? Converging evidence that self-esteem serves as an anxiety-buffering function. In: Baumeister RF (ed.) *The Self in Social Psychology*, Reading 6. Philadelphia, PA: Psychology Press.

Haley L, McKay EA (2004) 'Baking gives you the confidence': User's views of engaging in the occupation of baking. *British Journal of Occupational Therapy* 67(3):125–128.

Hewlett S (2003) Patients and clinicians have different perspective on outcomes in arthritis. *Journal of Rheumatology* 30(4):877–879.

Ilott I (1995) Occupational science: The foundation for practice. *British Journal of Therapy and Rehabilitation* 2(7):367–370.

Katz P (1995) The impact of rheumatoid arthritis on life activities. *Arthritis Care and Research* 8(4):272–278.

Keat AC, Gaffney K, Gillieri AK, et al. (2008) Influence of biologic therapy on return to work in people with work disability due to ankylosing spondylitis. *Rheumatology* 47:481–483.

Keilhofner G (2002) Doing and becoming: Occupational change and development. In: Keilhofner G (ed.) *Model of Human Occupation*. Baltimore, MD: Lippincott, Williams and Wilkins.

Kepnen R, Kielhofner G (2006) Occupation and meaning in the lives of women with chronic pain. *Scandinavian Journal of Occupational Therapy* 13:211–220.

Kielhofner G, ForsythK (1997) The model of human occupation: An overview of current concepts. *British Journal of Occupational Therapy* 60(3):103–110.

Knittle KP, de Gucht V, Hurkmans EJ, et al. (2011) Effect of self-efficacy and physical activity gaol achievement on arthritis pain and quality of life in patients with rheumatoid arthritis. *Arthritis Care and Research* 63(11):1613–1619.

Landa-Gonzalez B, Molnar D (2012) Occupational therapy intervention: Effects on self-care, performance, satisfaction, self-esteem/self-efficacy, and role functioning of older Hispanic females with arthritis. *Occupational Therapy in Health Care*. Early Online: 1–11.

Linden C, Bjorklund A (2010) Living with rheumatoid arthritis and experiencing everyday life with TNFα blockers. *Scandinavian Journal of Occupational Therapy* 17:326–334.

MacKinnon JR, Avison WR, McCain GA (1994) Rheumatoid arthritis, occupational profiles and psychological adjustment. *Journal of Occupational Science* 1(4):3–10.

Mattingley C (1991) The narrative nature of clinical reasoning. *American Journal of Occupational Therapy* 45(11):998–1005.

McArthur MA, Mason R (2012) Theory into practice: A model to facilitate the integration of CPD. In: Chia SH, Harrison D (eds.) *Tools for Continuing Professional Development*. London: Quay Books.

McArthur MA, Goodacre L, Birt L (2012) Exploring the experiences of occupational gain in patients with inflammatory arthritis receiving antiTNFα treatment. *British Society for Rheumatology Conference*, Glasgow, Scotland, UK.

Mishler EG (1984) *The Discourse of Medicine. Dialectics of Medical Interviews.* Norwood, NJ: Ablex Publishing Corporation.

National Institute for Clinical Excellence (NICE) (2009) *Rheumatoid Arthritis: The Management of Rheumatoid Arthritis in Adults. Clinical Guidelines 79.* http://www.nice.org.uk/nicemedia/. Accessed on 20 December 2011.

Nelson D (1987) Occupation: Form and performance. *The American Journal of Occupational Therapy* 42:633–641.

Oliver MM (1996) *Understanding Disability: From Theory to Practice.* Basingstoke, UK: Macmillan.

Ozgul A, Peker F, Taskaynatan MA, et al. (2006) Effects of ankylosing spondylitis on health-related quality and different aspects of social life in young patients. *Clinical Rheumatology* 25(2):168–174.

Parnell T, Wilding C (2010) Where an occupation-focussed philosophy can take occupational therapy? *Australian Occupational Therapy Journal* 57:345–348.

Persson D, Andersson I, Eklund M (2011) Defying aches and re-evaluating daily doing: Occupational perspectives on adjusting to pain. *Scandinavian Journal of Occupational Therapy* 18:188–197.

Rebeiro KL, Day D, Semeniuk B, et al. (2001) Northern initiative for social action: An occupation-based mental health program. *American Journal of Occupational Therapy* 55:493–500.

Reinseth L, Uhlig T, Kjeken I, et al. (2011) Performance in leisure-time physical activities and self-efficacy in females with rheumatoid arthritis. *Scandinavian Journal of Occupational Therapy* 18:210–288.

Schell BB (1998) Clinical reasoning: The basis of practice. In: Neistadt ME, Blesedell Crepeau E (eds.) *Willard and Spackman's Occupational Therapy.* Philadelphia, PA: Lippincott, Williams and Wilkins.

Schkade JK, Schulz S (1992) Occupational adaptation: Towards a holistic approach for contemporary practice, part 1. *American Journal of Occupational Therapy* 46:829–837.

Stamm T, Wright J, Machold K, et al. (2004) Occupational balance of women with rheumatoid arthritis: A qualitative study. *Musculoskeletal Care* 2(2):101–112.

Stamm T, Lovelock L, Stew G, et al. (2009) I have a disease but I am not ill: A narrative study of occupational balance in people with rheumatoid arthritis. *Occupational Therapy Journal of Research: Occupation, Participation and Health* 29(1):32–39.

Stephenson R (2012) Clinical reasoning as a tool for CPD. In: Chia SH, Harrison D (eds.) *Tools for Continuing Professional Development.* London: Quay Books.

Treichler PA, Frankel RM, Kramarae C, et al. (1987) Problems and problems: Power relationships in a medical encounter. In: Mayor BM, Pugh AK (eds.) *Language, Communication and Education.* London: Croom Helm in Association with the Open University.

Unruh AM (2004) So…what do you do? Occupation and the construction of identity. *Canadian Journal of Occupational Therapy* 71(5):290–295.

Unruh AM, Smith N, Scammell C (2000) The occupation of gardening in life-threatening illness: A qualitative pilot study. *Canadian Journal of Occupational Therapy* 67(2):70–77.

Vallacher RR, Wegner DM (1987) What do people think they're doing? Action identification and human behaviour. *Psychological Review* 94(1):3–15.

Vallacher RR, Wegner DM (1989) Levels of personal agency: Individual variation in action identification. *Journal of Personality and Social Psychology* 57(4):660–671.

Van Vollenhoven RF, Cifaldi MA, Ray S, et al. (2010) Improvement in work place and household productivity for patients with early rheumatoid arthritis treated with adalimumab plus methotrexate: Work outcomes and their correlations with clinical and radiographic measures from a randomized controlled trial companion study. *Arthritis Care and Research* 62(2):226–234.

Verstappen SMM, Watson KD, Lunt M (2010) Working status in patients with rheumatoid arthritis, ankylosing spondylitis and psoriatic arthritis: Results from the British Society for Rheumatology Biologics Register. *Rheumatology* 49:1570–1577.

Wagman P, Hakansson C, Bjorklund A (2012) Occupational balance as used in occupational therapy. *Scandinavian Journal of Occupational Therapy* 19(4):322–327.

Wilcock A (1995) The occupational brain: A theory of human nature. *Journal of Occupational Science* 2(1):68–73.

Wilcock AA (1998) *An Occupational Perspective of Health*. Thorofare, NJ: Slack.

Wilcock AA (1999) Reflections on doing, being and becoming. *Australian Journal of Occupational Therapy* 46:1–11.

Yelin E, Trupin L, Katz P, et al. (2003) Association between Etanercept use and employment outcomes among patients with rheumatoid arthritis. *Arthritis and Rheumatism* 48(11): 3046–3054.

Yerxa EJ, Clark F, Frank G, et al. (1990) An introduction to occupational science. A foundation for occupational therapy in the 21st century. *Occupational Therapy in Health Care* 6(4):1–17.

Chapter 4

Managing rheumatic conditions: the policy perspective

Lynne Goodacre

Lancaster University, Lancaster, United Kingdom

4.1 Introduction

The clinical management of people living with a rheumatic condition is located within a broad policy context which directly shapes health and social care agendas, resource allocation and clinical targets. Whilst on an individual level occupational therapists may prefer to focus on their clinical practice, such practice is inherently shaped and influenced by health and social care policy. It is therefore important to understand and engage with the broader policy context within which rheumatology occupational therapy is located and to understand at a personal and professional level our role in shaping and influencing policy.

Policy is of course dynamic and evolving and, within the context of devolution, will vary depending upon where in the United Kingdom (UK) a therapist is practicing. Therefore, this chapter will outline the key factors currently shaping health and social care in the UK and explore how these factors influence the management of people with long-term and rheumatic conditions. The chapter will provide an overview of the global challenges of meeting the needs of a growing ageing population living with an increasing burden of long-term conditions (LTCs) and explore how these two key factors are influencing and being addressed within the context of policies relevant to the management of long-term and rheumatic conditions.

4.2 Increase in the ageing population

Factors including the reduction in infectious diseases and improvements in health care, housing and sanitation have led to a significant increase in life expectancy on a

Rheumatology Practice in Occupational Therapy: Promoting Lifestyle Management, First Edition.
Edited by Lynne Goodacre and Margaret McArthur.
© 2013 John Wiley & Sons, Ltd. Published 2013 by John Wiley & Sons, Ltd.

global level. Whilst this is a positive trend to be welcomed, an increasingly ageing population poses a number of significant challenges, especially with regard to health and social care, housing, transport, workforce and pensions (Office for National Statistics 2012a). Whilst this global trend is well documented, it is worth pausing to contextualise this issue:

- Between 1985 and 2010, the number of people aged 65 and over in the UK increased by 20% to 10.3 million (Office for National Statistics 2012a).
- In 2010, 17% of the population was aged 65 and over. The same population will by 2035 account for 23% of the total population (2012a).
- Between 1985 and 2010, the number of people aged 85 and over more than doubled to 1.4 million. By 2035, this number is projected to reach 3.5 million (Office for National Statistics 2011a).
- Current projections suggest that the number of centenarians in the UK will exceed 160,000 by mid 2040. This would equate to more than a 12-fold increase from the 2010 figure (Office of National Statistics 2011b).
- Life expectancy in different regions of the UK varies by as much as 14 years (Office of National Statistics 2012b).
- As people born in the 1960s reach retirement age, they will be replaced in the working population by smaller numbers of people born since the 1960s, causing the ratio of retired people to those of working age to rise considerably, putting increased pressure on the pension system (Office of National Statistics 2012c).

Located within the context described previously, it is clear that the number of people with age-related rheumatic conditions like osteoarthritis (OA) will increase as will the number of people ageing with rheumatic conditions. Given this trend, significant emphasis is being placed, in policy terms, on ensuring that older people stay as healthy as possible for as long as possible and are engaged in and making a positive contribution to society. A key policy objective is therefore the promotion of active ageing.

Active ageing is defined as:

The process of optimizing opportunities for health, participation and security in order to enhance quality of life as people age (WHO 2002a).

Active ageing seeks to enable people to 'realize their potential for physical, social and mental well-being throughout their lives and to participate in society according to their needs, desires and capacities' (ESRC 2011). It is acknowledged that the promotion of active ageing is not only a health remit but is dependent upon what has been called a 'social-ecological' approach which encompasses evidence-based policy, community and neighbourhood action and individual interventions (Futurage 2011). Occupational therapists will be very familiar with the wide range of factors which influence participation, as reflected in this approach.

The success of this international policy objective will also be dependent upon an appreciation that active ageing is not something which begins at retirement age but is seen as a life-course objective which moves people away from a linear model of a life course which comprises stages of education, work and retirement and seeks to integrate all three across as much of the life course as possible (Futurage 2011). For example, education may take place across the life course as epitomised by the University of the Third Age (U3A) which seeks to promote shared learning for older people no longer in full-time work (U3A 2012). As the ratio of people over retirement age to those of working age increases, legislation is already in place to introduce a phased increase in the retirement age to 68 by 2046 with plans to speed up this change. Therefore, those in work will be required to work for longer before being eligible for state pension, but also it is recognised increasingly that people in work may choose to work beyond retirement age.

The role of occupational therapists in promoting active ageing has already been recognised through the work of Florence Clarke in the United States with regard to Lifestyle Redesign (Clarke et al. 2001) and Gail Mountain's work in the UK in the development of the Lifestyle Matters programme (Mountain et al. 2007). Whilst attention within active ageing has been focused on keeping the 'well elderly' well, in light of the significant increase in people ageing with a LTC, there is a need also to promote active ageing in the context of ageing with a LTC. The increasing challenge for occupational therapists working with older people with rheumatic conditions is that of developing interventions and promoting lifestyles which seek to ensure that they remain as healthy as possible for as long as possible.

4.3   Increase in long-term conditions

Alongside the increase in the ageing population, another key factor informing health and social care policy is the significant increase in the number of people living with at least one, and often more than one, LTC.

> A long-term condition is defined as 'a health problem which requires ongoing management over a period of years or decades' (WHO 2002b).

In 2008, the Department of Health published ten facts that need to be known about LTCs (Box 4.1), and, as with the statistics related to ageing, these are worth reflecting upon as they contextualise the size of the challenge facing health and social care services and also explain the significant policy focus on health promotion, the development of self-management skills and the proactive integrated approach to service design which seeks to prevent crisis and illness progression.

Whilst some of the statistics in Box 4.1 relate to England, the picture is the same across the UK with one third of all adults in Wales reporting having at least one LTC;

Box 4.1   Ten facts about long-term health conditions

1. In England, 15.4 million people (almost one in three of the population) have a LTC.
2. Three out of every five people aged over 60 in England have a LTC.
3. The number of people in England with a LTC is set to rise by 23% over the next 25 years.
4. Five per cent of clients, the majority of whom have one or more long-term condition, account for 49% of all inpatient hospital bed days.
5. Patients with LTCs account for 31% of the population but use 52% of all GP appointments and 65% of all outpatient appointments.
6. Estimates suggest that the treatment and care of people with LTCs accounts for 69% of the primary and acute care budget in England.
7. Estimates suggest that 6.4 million people have clinically identified hypertension. It is estimated that the same number again have unidentified hypertension, meaning that an estimated one in five of the population has the condition.
8. Common mental health problems affect about one in seven of the adult population with severe mental health problems affecting one in a hundred.
9. The UK economy stands to lose £16 billion over the next 10 years through premature deaths due to heart disease, stroke and diabetes.
10. It is estimated that 85% of deaths in the UK are from chronic diseases. Within this, 36% of all deaths will be from cardiovascular disease and 7% from chronic respiratory disease (DoH 2008).

---

an estimated two million people in Scotland live with a LTC, and in Northern Ireland the mortality rates for coronary heart disease are amongst the highest in Europe.

Given the significant economic costs associated with providing health and social care to people with LTCs, including the financing of welfare benefits and the costs associated with lost productivity, significant emphasis is being placed firstly on prevention, secondly on equipping those with LTCs with the knowledge, skills and confidence to play a central role in the self-management of their condition and thirdly on ensuring that services are configured to take a proactive integrated approach to the management of those with the most complex needs.

Promotion of effective management of people with long-term conditions

In 2004, the government's public health white paper, Choosing Health (DoH 2004), set out to address the underlying causes of LTC by promoting healthier lifestyle choices. This white paper was followed in 2005 by the publication of Supporting People with Long Term Conditions (DoH 2005a), which set out the strategic aim of embedding within health and social care 'an effective, systematic approach to the care and management of clients with a long term condition' (DoH 2005a, p. 5). Emphasis was placed on increasing care in the community and home environment, providing personalised care and equipping people with the knowledge and expertise to play an active role in their management of their impairment. The LTCs model set out a delivery system which was designed to ensure that people receive a level of care commensurate with the complexity of their needs. The model is conceptualised within three tiers (Figure 4.1):

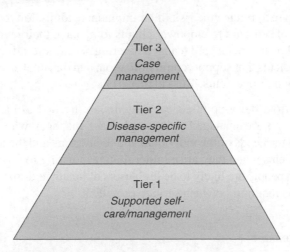

Figure 4.1 Generic long-term conditions model.

- Tier 1 is focused on acknowledging that clients, and their families, play a central role in the management of their conditions and ensuring that they are equipped with the skills, knowledge and expertise to manage their condition as effectively as possible.
- Tier 2 is focused on meeting the needs of those people who require a disease-specific approach to their management by promoting a proactive approach to management, which involves identifying needs early and responding promptly.
- Tier 3 is focused on meeting the needs of people with the most complex needs who utilise hospital and social care services regularly and are at risk of readmission.

The majority of people with rheumatic conditions will fall into tiers 1 and 2; however, some with more complex needs and multiple co-morbidities may require a case management approach.

Case management

Case management is focused on identifying those with complex multiple LTC and adopting a proactive integrated approach to their management. The delivery of effective case management is predicated upon being able to identify those in need of this level of support. A review by the Kings Fund (Ross et al. 2011) identified a range of factors important to the delivery of effective case management, which included:

- assigned accountability of an individual or team to provide continuity and a single line of responsibility for the care and services that a person receives,
- clarity about the role of the case managers and support to ensure they have the right clinical skills and managerial competencies,
- accurate case finding to ensure interventions are targeting those with defined care needs,
- appropriate caseloads to ensure that clients are receiving optimal care,
- a single point of access for assessment and a joint care plan,

- continuity of care to reduce the risk of an unplanned admission to hospital,
- the promotion of self-care to empower clients to manage their own conditions,
- integrated health and social care teams delivering services jointly and
- information systems that support communication, and data that are used proactively to drive quality improvements (Ross et al. 2011).

As can be seen from these points, clear systems are needed to identify those with complex needs who are managed by a single case manager who has an in-depth understanding of the needs of the individual and their carers and the ability to identify and resolve problems when they arise rather than responding to crisis if they are left unresolved. Such people are likely to be high users of health and social care, and good communication is required between service providers.

Disease management

Disease management is appropriate for people whose impairment is relatively under control and whose needs can be met via multidisciplinary team involvement through integrated services which span across primary and secondary care. The management of people with rheumatoid arthritis (RA), fibromyalgia and ankylosing spondylitis (AS) would fall into this category. The focus of this approach is on slowing progression, avoiding complications and reducing levels of disability (DoH 2005a), and is informed by following agreed pathways which incorporate regular review. The emphasis on regular review seeks to ensure, as with case management, that problems are identified early and acted upon to avoid unnecessary hospital admission and the need for crisis management. In many departments of rheumatology, people with rheumatic conditions have annual review appointments to monitor disease progression and highlight any factors which need to be addressed in terms of the impact of the impairment upon a person's quality of life.

Supported self-care and self-management

Supported self-care and self-management has been identified as being appropriate for 70–80% of people with LTCs (DoH 2005b), and it is important therefore to be clear about what these terms mean. Self-care has been described as 'the actions people take for themselves, their children and their families to stay fit and maintain good physical and mental health; meet social and psychological needs; prevent illness or accidents; care for minor ailments and long-term conditions; and maintain health and well-being after an acute illness or discharge from hospital' DoH (2005b).

Self-management is described as individuals 'making the most of their lives by coping with difficulties and making the most of what they have. It includes managing or minimising the way conditions limit individuals' lives as well as what they can do to feel happy and fulfilled to make the most of their lives despite the condition' (Skills for Health 2008).

Attention should be drawn to the use of the word 'supported' self-care and self-management, which highlights that this is a collaborative process undertaken by a person with a LTC and healthcare professionals. In 2008, Skills for Health published seven core principles which should inform the practice of healthcare professionals working with people with LTCs to support and promote self-care:

- Principle 1: Ensure individuals are able to make informed choices to manage their self-care needs.
- Principle 2: Communicate effectively to enable individuals to assess their needs, and develop and gain confidence to self-care.
- Principle 3: Support and enable individuals to access appropriate information to manage their self-care needs.
- Principle 4: Support and enable individuals to develop skills in self-care.
- Principle 5: Support and enable individuals to use technology to support self-care.
- Principle 6: Advise individuals how to access support networks and participate in the planning, development and evaluation of services.
- Principle 7: Support and enable risk management and risk taking.

These principles are relevant to the practice of rheumatology occupational therapists integrating self-management within their interventions. The focus of the interventions should be on facilitating and supporting the development of skills and expertise to enable people to manage their impairment with the reassurance that when/if necessary, they can call upon the expertise and support of relevant healthcare professionals.

Expert Patient Programme

Current approaches to the self-management of LTCs in the UK have been informed by the work of Lorig and colleagues in the United States, who, in the 1980s, developed the Arthritis Self-Management Programme. Evaluation of the Arthritis Self-Management Programme via a randomised controlled trial demonstrated that participants in the programme experienced a reduction in pain, improved quality of life and used fewer medical services (Lorig et al. 1993). Subsequent follow-up of participants in the trial suggested that these improvements were maintained for at least 4 years. The Arthritis Self-Management Programme was adopted in the UK by Arthritis Care and renamed the Challenging Arthritis Programme. Both of these programmes were underpinned by Bandura's work on self-efficacy, which is explored further in Chapter 7, and incorporated a range of techniques designed to increase self-efficacy and facilitate behaviour change.

The work of Lorig informed the development of the Expert Patient Programme (EPP), which was piloted in the UK between 2002 and 2004 and was developed as an integral component of the government's generic approach to the promotion of self-management for people with LTCs (DoH 2005a). In line with the theoretical emphasis of increasing self-efficacy, a central tenet of the EPP is the use of trained tutors, who have personal experience of living with a LTC, to deliver the course. The EPP is delivered via six weekly sessions and covers topics such as dealing with pain and fatigue, coping with feelings of depression, relaxation techniques, exercise, healthy eating, communicating with family, friends and healthcare professionals and planning for the future (Expert Patient Programme 2012).

In 2007, responsibility for the delivery of the EPP was transferred to a community interest company (CIC) whose purpose was described as 'establishing the principle of individual self-management and self-care as a recognised public health measure, deliverable in a cost effective and sustained way' (Expert Patient Programme 2012). Since its inception, the EPP CIC has increased the range of programmes offered to include courses for carers ('Looking After Me' and 'Supporting Parents and Young Carers') and young people ('Staying Positive', a course for 12–18 year olds living with a LTC). Whilst the generic EPP is still delivered, a range of condition-specific courses have also been developed related to substance and alcohol misuse, persistent pain, choosing self-management for life, diabetes, learning difficulties and recovering from or living with a mental health condition. The majority of these programmes are delivered face to face but the EPP is now also available online.

Educational approaches within departments of rheumatology

Alongside the EPP and the Arthritis Self-Management Programme, many departments of rheumatology develop their own educational programmes which are delivered on either an individual or group basis. For many rheumatology practitioners, education is a central component of their practice in terms of providing information and undertaking educational programmes designed to change behaviour.

Promotion of healthier lifestyles

Given the significant increase in LTCs, considerable resource is being put into primary prevention to avoid occurrence of disease in the first place, and secondary prevention to detect and treat disease early to prevent progression. The role of occupational therapists in health promotion is outlined within the College of Occupational Therapists publication, 'Health Promotion in Occupational Therapy' (COT 2008), which identifies it as one of the core skills of occupational therapists.

Health promotion has been described as encompassing 'health education, lifestyle and preventative approaches alongside the environmental, legal and fiscal measures designed to advance health' and occurring on three overlapping levels (Figure 4.2) (Scriven and Atwal 2004, p. 425).

Primary health promotion: is focused on the well population seeking to prevent ill health and disability, for example, campaigns targeting lifestyle and behavioural change such as the Change4Life (2012) campaign promoting healthier lifestyles (www.nhs.uk/change4life) and/or legislation, for example, the prohibition of smoking in public spaces.

Secondary health promotion: is focused on changing health-damaging habits, preventing ill health progressing and, where possible, restoring people to their former state of

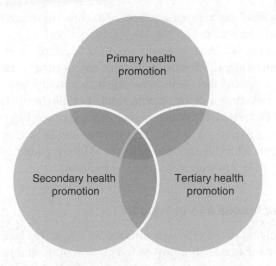

Figure 4.2 The long-term conditions model.

health, empowering people to take more control of their health and/or community development approaches which encourage structural and environmental changes.

Tertiary health promotion: is focused on working with individuals who have LTCs and/or are disabled to maximise their potential for healthy living.

Some programmes of primary health promotion will impact directly on seeking to reduce the incidence of rheumatic conditions; for example, obesity is recognised as one of the four most common problems linked with OA, and links have been established between obesity and the development of OA of the knee (Felson et al. 2000). Therefore, if the levels of obesity are reduced in the population, there should be a reduction in the population burden associated with OA.

Other programmes focusing on issues like smoking cessation, reducing drug misuse and alcohol consumption, the promotion of healthy diet and increasing physical activity may not impact directly on rheumatic conditions but could reduce the incidence of co-morbid conditions in people with rheumatic conditions. Both RA and AS are associated with increased rates of cardiovascular disease associated with an increased mortality (Goodson and Solomon 2006), and inactivity is associated with increased risk of coronary heart disease, OA and diabetes (Minor 1991).

Therefore, it is important for occupational therapists working with people with rheumatic conditions to understand the key public health challenges facing the population and to take every opportunity to explore and integrate health promotion messages into their daily practice, seeing every contact with a client as an opportunity to engage in health promotion.

Living with a rheumatic condition can make leading a healthier lifestyle more challenging as the levels of engagement in physical activity can be limited due to pain and fatigue, reduced self-confidence in engaging with exercise classes and groups, uncertainty about what is an appropriate level of exercise in which to engage and fear of making the condition worse.

However, increasing guidance is being provided to people with rheumatic conditions to enable them to identify forms of exercise appropriate to their specific impairment (Arthritis Care), and the concept of physical activity now embraces a wide range of activities including walking, dancing and Tai Chi (Brodin et al. 2008; Fransen et al. 2007). It is important for occupational therapists working with people with rheumatic conditions to understand the importance of their role in health promotion and in helping people with rheumatic conditions to interpret and adapt relevant guidance to the context of living with a rheumatic condition.

The integration of mental health support

In 2011, the publication of the cross-government strategy, 'No health without mental health', highlighted the need for improved integration of mental health services with primary care and long-term disease management (DoH 2011). A report from the Kings Fund has highlighted the significant impact and cost of poor mental health in people with LTCs, suggesting that the interaction between physical illness and co-morbid mental health problems increases the cost of health care by at least 45% for each person living with a LTC and co-existing mental health problem equating to between 12% and 18% of all expenditure on LTCs in England (Kings Fund 2012).

To locate the significance of this strategy to the context of people living with rheumatic conditions, the prevalence of depression in people with RA is estimated to be 13–20%, with people with RA being twice as likely to experience depression as members of the general population (Dickens and Creed 2001). Psychological distress is also reported by people with AS with studies suggesting that up to one third of people with AS experience depressive symptoms (Barlow 1993) and is a significant issue for people with fibromyalgia.

4.4   The delivery of efficient client-centred approaches to health and social care

A strong thread running through a range of health and social care policies is that of providing integrated services centred around the needs of client.

Integrated care

Many clients with rheumatic conditions will utilise a range of services provided through health, social care and voluntary sector. National Voices, a coalition of health and social care charities in England (National Voices 2012), and the Futures Forum (Goodwin et al. 2012) both identified the significant frustration that service users experience when services are not integrated. For client to have a positive experience, it is recognised that emphasis needs to be placed on the delivery of integrated care, which has been described as 'an approach that seeks to improve the quality of care for individual clients, service users and carers by ensuring that services are well co-ordinated around their needs' (Goodwin et al. 2012).

Having collected views and perspectives from a wide range of stakeholders, the Futures Forum (Goodwin et al. 2012) reported that a key element of integrated care is that it should be designed around clients, not around pathways, to ensure that meeting the needs of individuals is at the heart of service provision; care pathways by their generic approach are less able to do this.

client-centred approaches to working

> *Client-centred care* is defined as:
>
> Providing care that is respectful of and responsive to individual client preferences, needs, and values and ensuring that client values guide all clinical decisions (Institute of Medicine 2001).

Many of the characteristics of client-centred care expressed earlier are reflected in the Department of Health's description of a positive client experience, which has been described as:'...having information to make choices, to feel confident and feel in control; being talked to and listened to as an equal; and being treated with honesty, respect and dignity' (DoH 2005c).

Alongside defining client-centred care, the Institute for Medicine also outlined the different aspects of this approach:

- compassion, empathy and responsiveness to needs, values and expressed preferences,
- co-ordination and integration,
- information, communication and education,
- physical comfort,
- emotional support, relieving fear and anxiety and
- involvement of family and friends (Institute of Medicine 2001).

Within these dimensions, it is possible to identify areas of synergy with the increased emphasis on self-management described earlier, which seeks to ensure that people feel more informed about and in control of the management of their impairment, alongside the development of integrated service.

The description of a positive client experience also highlights other areas of policy focus such as 'making choices', articulated in the White Paper Equity and Excellence: Liberating the NHS (DoH 2010) as 'shared decision-making will become the norm: no decision about me without me'. This means ensuring that clients are equipped with information about the range of potential treatment options and choices open to them and that they are supported in playing an active role in making informed decisions about their treatment and care. The level of support required will vary from person to person, but a clear emphasis is now placed on ensuring that shared decision making is a part of routine practice.

Similar policy initiatives are also taking place with regard to social care located within the personalisation agenda which seeks to place the person at the centre of decision making about their care, enabling them to agree a plan of how that care will be delivered. The Social Care Institute for Excellence describes the key dimensions of personalisation as:

- tailoring support to individuals needs,
- ensuring that people have access to information, advocacy and advice to make informed decisions about their care,
- finding new ways of working collaboratively to enable people to engage actively in the design, delivery and evaluation of services,
- developing local partnerships to co-produce services for people to choose from and opportunities for social inclusion and community development,
- developing leadership and organisational systems to enable staff to work in person-centred ways,
- embedding early intervention, re-ablement and prevention to support people early,
- recognising and supporting carers while enabling them to maintain their own life and
- ensuring that everyone has access to universal community services and resources (Carr 2008).

4.5   Shaping policy to meet the needs of people with rheumatic conditions

The preceding sections of this chapter have highlighted key factors which are currently informing and will continue to inform health and social care for some time to come. Whilst policy is determined by government and enacted by service providers, it is not formulated within a vacuum but is informed by the views and experiences of key stakeholder groups. Many of the leading organisations representing people with rheumatic conditions such as The National Ankylosing Spondylitis Society, UK Fibromyalgia, Arthritis Care and National Rheumatoid Arthritis Society as well as professional bodies such as the College of Occupational Therapists and the British Society for Rheumatology undertake a range of influencing activities to inform policy.

Such organisations are increasingly working together to exert more power, and a key umbrella organisation working on behalf of people with rheumatic conditions is the Arthritis and Musculoskeletal Alliance (ARMA), which was founded with the mission of 'transforming the quality of life for people with musculoskeletal disorders' with a specific focus on shaping policy and best practice (ARMA 2012). Alongside engaging in influencing policy, ARMA has developed a range of standards of care which provide a framework for services with people with rheumatic conditions and encompass standards for inflammatory arthritis, OA, back pain and regional musculoskeletal pain. The standards provide benchmarks against which services can be audited, and ARMA has developed audit tools to facilitate this process.

4.6 Conclusions

Health and social care policy is a changing landscape which has a significant impact upon the practice of occupational therapists and the services and support available to people living with rheumatic conditions. Many occupational therapists will experience the impact of policy within their clinical practice at differing levels and may be responsible for delivering policy agendas. Rather than seeing policy as something which is reacted to the potential for individuals and organisations to influence and shape policy should also be considered by responding to relevant consultations via the College of Occupational Therapists or other representative bodies such as British Healthcare Professionals in Rheumatology or taking up a place on the wide range of committees which influence policy agendas.

Resources

Websites

Arthritis and Musculoskeletal Alliance – Containing standards for care and other policy information relevant to people with rheumatic conditions. http://armu. uk.net/resources/. Accessed on 20 November 2012.

e-Learning for Healthcare. http://www.e-lfh.org.uk/projects/supportingselfcare/index. html. Accessed on 14 November 2012.

Kings Fund. www.kingsfund.org.uk. Accessed on 14 November 2012.

Long-Term Conditions Alliance Northern Ireland. http://www.ltcani.org.uk/. Accessed on 14 November 2012.

Long-Term Conditions Alliance Scotland. http://www.alliance-scotland.org.uk. Accessed on 20 November 2012.

Selfmanagement.co.uk, a resource comprising self-management resources, news, information and advice about all aspects of self-management of long-term health conditions. www.selfmanagement.co.uk/front. Accessed on 14 November 2012.

Social Care Institute for Excellence. http://www.scie.org.uk/Index.aspx. Accessed on 14 November 2012.

References

Arthritis and Musculoskeletal Alliance (ARMA) (2012). http://arma.uk.net/. Accessed on 12 January 2012.

Barlow J, Macey S, Struthers G (1993) Gender, depression and ankylosing spondylitis. *Arthritis Care and Research* 6(1):45–51.

Brodin N, Eurenius E, Jensen I, et al. (2008) Coaching patients with early rheumatoid arthritis to healthy physical activity: A multi-centre, randomized, controlled study. *Arthritis and Rheumatism* 59(3):325–331.

Carr S (2008) *Personalisation a Rough Guide Social Care Institute for Excellence Guide 47*. http://www.scie.org.uk/publications/guides/guide47/index.asp. Accessed on 19 February 2012.

Change4Life. www.nhs.uk/change4life. Accessed on 12 January 2012.

Clarke F, Stanley P, Azen R, et al. (2001) Embedding health promotion changes into the lives of independent living older adults: Long term follow up of an occupational therapy intervention. *Journal of Gerontology: Psychological Sciences* 56B(1):60–63.

College of Occupational Therapists (COT) (2008) *Health Promotion in Occupational Therapy*. London: College of Occupational Therapists. Dickens C, Creed F (2001) The burden of depression in patients with rheumatoid arthritis. *Rhuematology* 40(12):1327–1330.

Department of Health (DoH) (2004) *Choosing Health. Making Healthy Choices Easier*. London: Department of Health.

DoH (2005a) *Supporting People with Long Term Conditions*. London: Department of Health.

DoH (2005b) *Self Care – A Real Choice*. London: Department of Health.

DoH (2005c) *Now I Feel Tall. What a Patient Led NHS Feels Like*. London: Department of Health.

DoH (2008) *Ten Things You Need to Know about Long Term Conditions NHS*. London: Department of Health. http://webarchive.nationalarchives.gov.uk/+/www.dh.gov.uk/en/Healthcare/Longtermconditions/DH_084294. Accessed on 19 February 2012.

DoH (2010) *Equity and Excellence: Liberating the NHS*. London: Department of Health.

DoH (2011) *No Health without Mental Health: A Cross-Government Mental Health Outcomes Strategy for People of All Ages*. London: Department of Health.

Economic and Social Research Council (ESRC) (2011) *Independence Crucial to Wellbeing in Older Age*. London: ESRC Evidence Briefing. http://www.esrc.ac.uk/_images/Wellbeing%20in%20older%20age_tcm8-18760.pdf. Accessed on 12 January 2012.

Expert Patient Programme (2012). http://www.expertpatients.co.uk/. Accessed on 12 January 2012.

Felson DT, Lawrence RC, Dieppe PA, et al. (2000) Osteoarthritis: New insights. Part 1: The disease and its risk factors. *Annals of Internal Medicine* 133(8):635–646.

Fransen M, Nairn L, Winstanley J, et al. (2007) Physical activity for osteoarthritis management: A randomized controlled clinical trial evaluating hydrotherapy or Tai Chi classes. *Arthritis Care & Research* 57:407–414.

Futurage (2011) *A Road Map for European Ageing Research University of Sheffield*. London: Futurage. http://futurage.group.shef.ac.uk/road-map.html. Accessed on 12 January 2012.

Goodson N, Solomon D (2006) The cardiovascular manifestations of rheumatic diseases. *Current Opinion in Rheumatology* 18:135–140.

Goodwin N, Smith J, Davies A, et al. (2012) *Integrated Care for Patients and Populations: Improving Outcomes by Working Together*. A report to the Department of Health and the NHS Future Forum 2012. http://www.kingsfund.org.uk/publications/integrated-care-patients-and-populations-improving-outcomes-working-together. Accessed on 19 February 2012.

Institute of Medicine (2001) *Crossing the Quality Chasm: A New Health System for the 21st Century*. Washington, DC: National Academy Press.

Kings Fund (2012) *Long-Term Conditions and Mental Health: The Cost of Co-Morbidities.* London: The King's Fund. http://www.kingsfund.org.uk/document.rm?id=9438. Accessed on 12 January 2012.

Lorig KR, Mazonson PD, Holman HR (1993) Evidence suggesting that health education for self-management in patients with chronic arthritis has sustained health benefits while reducing health care costs. *Arthritis and Rheumatism* 36(4):439–446.

Minor M (1991) Physical activity and the management of arthritis. *Annals of Behavioural Medicine* 13:117–124.

Mountain G, Mozley C, Craig C, et al. (2007) Occupational therapy led health promotion for older people: Feasibility of the lifestyle matters programme. *British Journal of Occupational Therapy* 71(10):406–413.

National Voices (2012) *Integrated Care: What Do Patients, Service Users and Carers Want.* London: National Voices. www.nationalvoices.org.uk/sites/www.nationalvoices.org.uk/files/what_patients_want_from_integration_national_voices_paper.pdf. Accessed on 12 January 2012.

Office for National Statistics (2011a) *Older People in the UK.* London. Office for National Statistics. http://www.ons.gov.uk/ons/rel/mortality-ageing/focus-on-older-people/older-people-s-day-2011/stb-opd-2011.html#tab-Older-people-in-the-UK. Accessed on 19 February 2012.

Office for National Statistics (2011b) *Estimates of Centenarians in the UK.* London: Office for National Statistics. http://www.ons.gov.uk/ons/rel/mortality-ageing/population-estimates-of-the-very-elderly/2010/sum-eve 2010.html. Accessed on 19 February 2012.

Office for National Statistics (2012a) *Topic Guide to Older People.* London: Office for National Statistics. http://www.statistics.gov.uk/hub/population/ageing/older-people. Accessed on 19 February 2012.

Office for National Statistics (2012b) *Pension Trends: Life Expectancy and Healthy Ageing.* London: Office for National Statistics. http://www.ons.gov.uk/ons/rel/pensions/pension-trends/chapter-3–life-expectancy-and-healthy-ageing–2012-edition-/index.html. Accessed on 19 February 2012.

Office for National Statistics (2012c) *Pension Trends: Population Change.* London: Office for National Statistics. http://www.ons.gov.uk/ons/rel/pensions/pension-trends/chapter-2–population-change–2012-edition-/index.html. Accessed on 19 February 2012.

Ross S, Curry N, Goodwin N (2011) *Case Management. What It Is and How It Can Best Be Implemented.* London: The King's Fund. www.kingsfund.org.uk/publications/case_management.html. Accessed on 14 November 2012.

Scriven A, Atwal A (2004) Occupational therapists as primary health promoters: Opportunities and barriers. *British Journal of Occupational Therapy* 67(10):424–429.

Skills for Health (2009) *Common Core Principles to Support Self-Care.* London: Skills for Care Ltd. http://www.skillsforhealth.org.uk/component/docman/doc_view/1485-self-care-main-report.html. Accessed on 19 February 2012.

University of the Third Age (U3A) (2012). http://www.u3a.org.uk/. Accessed on 19 February 2012.

World Health Organization (WHO) (2002a) *Active Ageing. A Policy Framework.* Geneva, Switzerland: WHO.

WHO (2002b) *Innovative Care for Chronic Conditions: Building Blocks for Action.* Geneva, Switzerland: WHO.

Chapter 5

Occupational therapy assessment and outcome measurement

Annette Sands[1] and Lynne Goodacre[2]

[1]*Wrightington, Wigan and Leigh NHS Foundation Trust, Wigan, United Kingdom;*
[2]*Lancaster University, Lancaster, United Kingdom*

5.1 Introduction

Accurate and timely assessment is fundamental to the occupational therapy process and enshrined within the College of Occupational Therapists (COT) code of ethics and professional conduct, which states that 'the duty of care would require you to assess the suitability of the potential service user for occupational therapy with reasonable care and skill following usual and approved occupational therapy practice' (COT 2010). The Professional Standards for Occupational Therapy Practice (COT 2011) also contains five standards statements relating to assessment and goal setting. Taken together, these documents firmly locate assessment as a core component and requirement of occupational therapists.

In this chapter, we will explore the factors which influence the choice of assessment, provide an overview of the assessment process and relevant data-collection tools and emphasise the importance of integrating outcome measurement into the assessment process.

The following definitions of assessment and outcome measurement will be adopted throughout this chapter:

Assessment

The overall *process of selecting* and using *multiple data-collection tools* and various sources of information to inform decisions required for guiding therapeutic intervention during the whole therapy process. It involves interpreting information collected to make clinical decisions related to the needs of the person and the appropriateness and nature of their therapy (Laver-Fawcett 2007, p. 5).

Rheumatology Practice in Occupational Therapy: Promoting Lifestyle Management, First Edition.
Edited by Lynne Goodacre and Margaret McArthur.
© 2013 John Wiley & Sons, Ltd. Published 2013 by John Wiley & Sons, Ltd.

The phrases 'the process of selection' and the use of 'multiple data-collection tools' convey the active role played by therapists in determining the assessments they use and the utilisation of several data-collection tools in the assessment process. Therapists therefore need to be conversant with a range of tools and develop an understanding of how to select the most appropriate tool for a specific purpose.

Outcome measurement

A process undertaken to *establish the effects of an intervention* on an individual *or the effectiveness of a service* on a *defined aspects* of the health or well being of a specific population. Outcome measurement is achieved by administering an outcome measure on at *least two occasions* to document *change over time*…(Laver-Fawcett 2007, p. 12).

Outcome measurement therefore involves the administration of an appropriate measure as part of the process of assessment. If a standardised assessment is used on one occasion, it is a tool for data collection which can inform treatment planning, and if it is used at the beginning and end of an intervention, it also becomes an outcome measure with the ability to measure the effectiveness an intervention.

5.2   Outcome measurement: the policy context

Whilst the earlier definitions of assessment and outcome measurement emphasise their role in informing decisions to guide clinical decision making, it is important to locate outcome measurement within the wider policy context in which occupational therapy services are provided.

The outcomes agenda

The government's stated intention to drive a 'relentless focus on clinical outcomes' (DoH 2010) has increased the need to think about the ways in which the outcomes of interventions can be demonstrated. The utilisation of standardised assessments is essential to produce robust evidence against nationally agreed goals (DoH 2010; NHS Scotland 2010; Welsh Government 2011) which demonstrate improvements in the quality and efficiency of service delivery.

Patient reported outcomes

Set alongside the requirement to demonstrate the clinical outcomes of interventions is the requirement to demonstrate outcomes in terms of 'results that really matter to clients' (DoH 2010). Such outcomes are frequently assessed via Patient Reported Outcome Measures (PROMs) which are typically self-completed questionnaires administered to people to assess their self-reported health status or quality of life (DoH 2008). For example, since 2009 it has been a requirement of all licensed providers of unilateral hip and knee replacements to collect PROMs (DoH 2009) using the Oxford Hip (Dawson et al. 1996) and Oxford Knee scores (Dawson et al. 1998). The focus on collecting client reported outcomes is an acknowledgement that clients and healthcare professionals may have different perspectives about what is a good outcome (Carr et al. 2003; Hewlett 2003; Hewlett et al. 2001) and that clients' perspectives are central in informing service delivery and development.

Shared decision making

The aim of involving clients more fully in decisions about their health care has been articulated as 'Nothing about me without me' (DoH 2010). Client-centred working has always been central to occupational therapy practice but when applied to the assessment process requires therapists to ensure that the process captures domains of importance to clients so that when priorities for intervention are identified clients have the ability to play an active role in not only identifying areas of concern but also in informing treatment decisions.

5.3   The occupational therapy assessment process

Whilst the policy context influences the assessment process, assessment should be driven by the need to inform clinical decisions. Within the context of working with people with rheumatic conditions, assessment may take place in relation to a single intervention or, given the long-term nature of many rheumatic conditions, form an ongoing component of a therapeutic relationship. In such an instance, assessment is an ongoing, fluid process that facilitates monitoring of treatment progress and refocusing and reprioritising of treatment goals and interventions, particularly during periods of exacerbation and remission.

The initial stage of the assessment process usually begins with a referral outlining the problem with which a person is presenting. The source and format of the referral will vary depending on the context within which a therapist is working. Within a hospital context, it may provide clinical information such as joint involvement, systemic symptoms, pain and fatigue; within a community setting, it may be more activity focused, outlining a specific area of activity limitation. Within either setting, referral may focus on an intervention, e.g. promoting self-management, splinting. Whichever format it takes, the referral triggers the start of an assessment informed by the information-gathering process of the initial interview, the structure and duration of which will vary according to the reason for referral.

In some clinical centres, it forms part of a larger multi-disciplinary team (MDT) assessment during which a person sees all members of the team on one visit with agreements amongst team members about which aspects of assessment they will focus upon. Information is then shared across the team to inform treatment planning. Alternatively, one member of the MDT may carry out the initial assessment and identify areas for treatment which are then referred to the appropriate team member;

this occurs predominantly in MDT review clinics. In other settings, the occupational therapist will be working alone and is responsible for gathering all of the relevant information to inform interventions.

The initial interview therefore provides the first opportunity to gain a comprehensive understanding of the problems, concerns and limitations of a person and also to learn more about the wider context of their lives, focusing on strengths as well as limitations, priorities as well as problems. It may be conducted solely on the basis of a narrative interview or comprise a narrative interview and the use of standardised assessments.

Timing and duration

Taking part in a comprehensive initial interview can take time and for some people requires a great deal of concentration. Therapists should be aware of the impact of fatigue and stiffness on the interview process and the point at which two shorter interviews may be more appropriate.

If formal assessments are integrated into the interview, the time of day at which an assessment is conducted may affect the results. For example, if a person is required to perform a timed task at 9.00am, their performance may be affected by morning stiffness. It would therefore be important to conduct any follow-up assessment at the same time of the day to increase the reliability of the assessment as a change in result may be due to the timing of the assessment rather than the intervention.

Setting

The majority of occupational therapy assessments will take place within a clinical setting, the person's home or place of work. Whatever the setting, a confidential area free from interruption is necessary. Assessments carried out in a clinical environment may not be representative of the person's true abilities as their home or work environment cannot usually be simulated in a clinical environment. The impact of environmental challenges therefore needs to be taken into consideration during the assessment.

Involvement of others

Partners or other family members can be an important source of information; however, decisions need to be taken as to whether the inclusion of others is relevant and, if so, how this should be undertaken. This will depend on the purpose and nature of the assessment and whether it will be beneficial to obtain information from another individual; it may be appropriate to involve others if they are involved in the care arrangements for that person. Although there are potential benefits in involving others, there are also potential limitations; the person being assessed may be more inhibited, less communicative or more anxious. The issues of professional ethics and confidentiality must be considered, and any involvement that others have in a client's assessment should be based firmly on the wishes of the client.

5.4 Commonly used data-collection tools

The COT Specialist Section in Rheumatology Practice Guidelines (COT 2003) state that 'the occupational therapist evaluates clients using interviews, observations and formal standardised assessments', and these will be considered in more detail. However, before any assessment is undertaken, two questions need to be answered:

- Why am I undertaking this assessment? (the purpose)
- What do I need to assess? (the focus)

The answer to these questions will inform the way in which the assessment is carried out and the data-collection tools chosen as illustrated in Table 5.1.

In many instances, there will be a number of reasons requiring the use of a combination of data-collection tools; a clear rationale should always inform the choice of data-collection tool.

An occupational focus

If the evidence base for occupational therapy is to continue to develop a key factor, informing the choice of data-collection tool should be its relevance to occupation. The COT Professional standards define the purpose of occupational therapy as being, 'to enable people to fulfil, or to work towards fulfilling, their potential as occupational beings' (COT 2011). Therefore, whichever assessment tools are chosen, it is arguable that amongst them should be one with an occupational focus. For example, if the primary purpose of an intervention is to reduce fatigue, within the assessment there should be a focus not only determining the impact of the intervention on the severity and duration of fatigue but also of its impact on a person's ability to undertake and engage in meaningful occupations.

Table 5.1 Link between rationale for undertaking assessment and choice of data-collection tool.

Purpose	Data-collection tool
Establishing baseline information to inform clinical interventions	Referral Narrative interview Standardised assessment Observation
Developing an understanding of the wider contexts of a person's life	Narrative interview
Identifying priorities of clients to inform clinical decisions	Standardised assessment containing client preferencing Narrative interview
Monitoring disease progression over time	Standardised assessment
Determining the efficacy of an intervention	Standardised assessment

Narrative interviews

Narratives have been described as, 'the stories that people tell about themselves to give order to their lives' (Fox et al. 2007, p. 16) and, within the clinical context, are often used during the initial interview. Whilst the focus may be primarily on information gathering, the power of personal narrative has the potential to inform the therapeutic relationship. By providing a person with the space and time to 'tell their story', an opportunity can be provided for someone to make sense and meaning of what is happening to them (Greenhalgh and Hurwitz 1999). Narrative, as a client-centred approach, can give insights into aspects of a person's lived experience and thus inform treatment planning.

The narrative interview is usually semi-structured with at least several questions planned in advance which are open-ended and allow for sharing. It should provide an insight into how the person perceives themselves in various roles at home and work and during leisure time, how they respond to rest, activity, quality of sleep and any aggravating factors. Asking them to describe the pattern of their condition over the last 24 h can give insight into how they are coping. The client should be encouraged to speak freely about problems, concerns, troubles or interests. Components of their mental, physical and psychosocial performance should also be explored. This is particularly useful in those who have been recently diagnosed. Some notes should be taken; however, this should be explained as note taking can make some people uncomfortable and distract from the process. The interview should lead to the identification of areas of limitations and conclude with a discussion related to how these are going to be addressed in terms of proposed interventions.

Observational assessment

This involves the observed performance of tasks and may be those with which a person is less satisfied with their performance, e.g. opening jars/bottles or getting in/out of the bath. Depending on the task and rationale for undertaking the observation, the task may be carried out within a clinical setting or within a person's home or workplace. Observation within the environment in which the activity is carried out will provide a more accurate assessment (Table 5.2).

Table 5.2 Observational assessment.

Purpose	Advantages and limitations
To establish the client's level of independence, methods used in carrying out a task and the amount of stress and strain exerted on joints in the completion of the task	*Advantages*: provides direct access to the task under consideration. The choice of task is informed by the initial interview and more specific to the client. The occupational therapist can obtain information that might otherwise be difficult to assess accurately and can respond to events as they occur throughout the assessment such as advising on joint protection methods
	Limitations: Can be time consuming to observe a number of tasks. Informal observational assessment has been found to be less reliable than using measurement instruments (Myers et al. 2011). There is the potential for the observer to record what they thought they saw and not what actually happened

Examples

A specific activity can be set up for the person to perform, e.g. making a hot drink or getting out of the bath. By observing the areas of difficulty, e.g. difficulty with motor skills when filling the kettle, it is then possible to formulate a meaningful plan of intervention.

Standardised assessments

Whilst narrative-based interviews are deeply embedded within occupational therapist practice, the same is not true for the use of standardised assessments and the routine collection of outcome data with many therapists preferring to use locally based non-standard assessments (Hammond 1996). Whilst such assessments may provide detailed insights into clients' problems, they do not provide reliable and valid outcome data.

Standardised assessments have undergone a rigorous process of development and evaluation to ensure that they produce accurate and reliable information with the ability to detect change when change has occurred. There are many different types of standardised assessment, and Tables 5.3, 5.4, 5.5, 5.6 and 5.8 provide examples of commonly used assessments encompassing standardised observational assessment as well as generic, disease-specific, dimension-specific, population-specific and patient-generated assessments.

Standardised structured observational assessments

Table 5.3 Standardised structured observational assessments.

Purpose	Advantages and limitations
To measure performance in carrying out a specific task(s)	*Advantages*: a tightly, structured standardised approach enabling subsequent comparisons to be made across time. Allows for comparisons of outcomes between clients, treatment interventions and services
	Limitations: may not have access to the relevant equipment or be able to apply it in the clinical setting

Examples

The Sequential Occupational Dexterity Assessment (SODA) is validated for use with clients with rheumatoid arthritis (RA) and is designed to measure bi-manual dexterity in daily life (Van Lankveld et al. 1996). Twelve standardised unilateral and bilateral tasks are performed and the person is scored on their ability to perform them. Another standardised assessment used to assess hand strength and dexterity in adults with RA and osteoarthritis is the Arthritis Hand Function Test (Backman et al. 1991), which comprises 11 unilateral and bilateral tasks that are observed and timed.

Generic assessments

Table 5.4   Generic assessments.

Purpose	Advantages and limitations
To measure a number of dimensions identified as contributing to health and well-being	*Advantages*: suitable for use across a range of health problems and can therefore be used to compare interventions across different client groups. For example, in a community setting, an occupational therapist could use the SF36 with all clients and be able to understand the impact of the service as a whole
	Limitations: Because of their generic nature they can be less sensitive to the needs of specific client populations and therefore be less sensitive to picking up clinical improvement or deterioration

Examples

The EQ-5D is a generic measure of health status (EuroQol 1990) used widely in clinical trials, population studies and studies which seek to undertake an economic appraisal of an intervention. The Short Form-36 (SF36) (Ware and Sherbourne 1992) measures health status across eight domains: physical functioning, social functioning, role limitations due to physical problems, role limitations due to emotional problems, mental health, vitality, pain and general health perceptions. Both measures have undergone extensive evaluation (Table 5.4).

Disease-specific assessments

Table 5.5   Disease-specific assessments.

Purpose	Advantages and limitations
To measure a range of dimensions in specific client populations	*Advantages*: Being designed for use with specific populations the questions focus on issues relevant to that population. This makes the assessments more sensitive than generic instruments and also potentially more acceptable to clients as they understand the relevance of the questions
	Limitations: Because of their specificity they cannot be used across different client populations to derive data across a service

Examples

Therapists working within rheumatology have access to a wide range of disease-specific measures with varying degrees of specificity. The Arthritis Impact Measurement Scale (Meenan et al. 1992) was developed to measure health status in people with 'arthritis' assessing physical function, pain, psychological status, social interactions and support, health perceptions and treatment and demographic information. Other measures including the Fibromyalgia Impact Questionnaire (FIQ) (Burkhardt et al. 1991), which measures function, symptoms and the overall impact of fibromyalgia, and The EASI-Qol (Haywood et al. 2010), which measures quality of life in people with AS, have been developed for people with specific conditions (Table 5.5).

Dimension-specific assessments

Table 5.6 Dimension specific.

Purpose	Advantages and limitations
To measure a specific aspect of health	*Advantages*: Due to the focus on a specific dimension, the assessment will tend to be more detailed and more sensitive to detecting change. Their use will usually be informed by an initial interview which has identified a specific area of limitation/need
	Limitations: Their specific focus means they may be less useful in identifying a broad range of problems

Examples

The range of potential dimensions have been summarised by Garratt et al. (2002) as including physical function (e.g. hand function, mobility, activities of daily living), symptoms, global judgement of health, psychological well-being, social well-being, cognitive functioning, role activities (e.g. employment), personal constructs (e.g. satisfaction with bodily appearance) and satisfaction with care. Examples include the McGill Pain Questionnaire (Melzack 1975), which comprises four subscales measuring the affective, sensory, evaluative and miscellaneous aspects of pain, and the Health Assessment Questionnaire (Fries et al. 1982), one of the most commonly used measures of functional status. The Arthritis Self-Efficacy Scale (Lorig et al. 1989) was developed to measure clients' beliefs that they could perform specific tasks to cope with the consequences of their condition and the Patient Health Questionnaire-9 (Spitzer et al. 1999) was developed to measure depression (Table 5.6).

Population-specific assessments

Table 5.7 Population specific.

Purpose	Advantages and limitations
To be used with a specific population such as children or older people	*Advantages*: As with disease-specific measures population-specific measures may have more relevance if working with a specific population with a range of different pathologies
	Limitations: May be less sensitive to the needs of people with specific conditions within the population

Example

For therapists working with adults with rheumatological conditions, population measures may be used less frequently than disease or dimension-specific measures as most therapists would be working with a generic caseload. However, there may be occasions when therapists are working with a specific population, such as older people, and feel it more appropriate to select an assessment developed specifically for the population. An example is the Older Persons Quality of Life Questionnaire (Bowling 2009) (Table 5.7).

Patient-generated assessments

Table 5.8   Patient-generated assessments.

Purpose	Advantages and limitations
To identify and measure dimensions identified as important by the client	*Advantages*: can be used to inform person centred practice *Limitations*: Usually administered as part of an interview process and therefore can take longer to complete. Can be more difficult to interpret across a client population

Example

Patient-generated assessments vary from those described previously as they do not comprise a list of predetermined questions to which a person responds. They have a structure and a standardised process of administration which leads to the generation, by each client, of a list of areas of concern which are then prioritised to inform treatment planning. The most widely used individualised questionnaire for occupational therapist would be the Canadian Occupational Performance Measure (Law et al. 1990), an assessment centred around shared decision making as therapist and client work together to identify areas of concern and priorities for intervention (Table 5.8).

5.5   Factors influencing the choice of data-collection tool

When assessment is located within the policy context outlined previously and combined with clinically related needs, it should become clear that no single data-collection tool could possibly meet all requirements. It should also be clear that an overreliance on the use of non-standardised assessment located within a narrative framework will meet few of the policy objectives leaving occupational therapy practice exposed and continuing to lack an evidence base. Therapists therefore need to become adept at understanding the contribution of different approaches to assessment and how

Table 5.9 Measures used by Macedo et al. (2009).

	Rationale for use	Mode of assessment
Primary outcome measure		
Canadian Occupational Performance Measure (Law et al. 1990)	To detect change in self-perception of occupational performance in terms of satisfaction with ability to perform and performance of client-identified areas of function	Interview-based assessment
Secondary outcome measures		
Health Assessment Questionnaire (Fries et al. 1982)	Measure of physical function	Self-complete questionnaire
The RA Work Instability Scale (Gilworth et al. 2003)	Screening tool for work disability	Self-complete questionnaire
Subscales of the Arthritis Impact Measurement Scale II (Meenan et al. 1992)	Measure mood, tension and pain	Self-complete questionnaire
The Arthritis Helplessness Index (Stein et al. 1988)	Measure self-perception of helplessness	Self-complete questionnaire
The EuroQol (EQ-5D) (Euroqol Group 1990)	Classify a person's health state	Self-complete questionnaire
Measures of disease activity		
Visual analogue scales for pain, fatigue, stiffness	Measure levels of pain, fatigue, stiffness	Self-complete questionnaire
Disease activity score (DAS 28) (Prevoo et al. 1995)	Measure current disease activity of RA	Clinical measurement and client global assessment

a number of tools can be integrated into practice in a way which does not place a significant burden on the assessment process in terms of time and resource for the client or therapist. This approach is illustrated within the context of a study undertaken to determine if a targeted, comprehensive occupational therapy intervention for people with RA:

(a) improved occupational performance
(b) resulted in improvements in physical function, work productivity, coping or disease activity.

(Macedo et al. 2009)

Having identified the focus of the intervention, a range of measures were identified to capture specific outcomes (Table 5.9).

We are not suggesting that in a clinical context such a range of measures would be used in one intervention, but this illustrates how the primary focus of an intervention should drive the choice of outcome measure and how multiple measures can be combined to assess different aspects of an intervention.

Choosing standardised assessment tools

The development and refinement of a standardised assessment takes place over a number of years with early work determining the content and the psychometric properties of the tool. Subsequent work will explore how sensitive the assessment is to change, its use in different client populations and what level of change in a score is required to indicate that a clinically important change has taken place. For some tools, ongoing development can lead to the development of a shorter version. Examples include the SF36 (Ware and Sherbourne 1992), which has been refined to produce the shorter SF12 (Ware et al. 1996), and SF6 (Ware et al. 2001) or the McGill Pain Questionnaire from which a short-form version has been produced (Melzack 1987). There are a number of different factors which should influence your choice of standardised assessment and these are described next.

Who was involved in developing the assessment?

As we have noted, there is significant emphasis on patient-reported outcomes, and it is helpful to understand the extent to which an assessment is client centred. A distinction can be made between assessments in which client have played a central role in informing the questions, e.g. the Measure of Activity Limitation (Goodacre et al. 2007), and assessments in which items have been derived from the views of healthcare professionals.

Another issue which can be established by going back to the original publication is the study population involved. This will help to determine if the assessment is relevant for the population with whom you are proposing to use it. For example, a measure may have been developed with clients with a long disease duration and you may be seeking an assessment to use with clients who are newly diagnosed. The assessment may be psychometrically strong but may not ask questions of relevance to a newly diagnosed population.

How much confidence can I have in the assessment?

The answer to this question requires an understanding of the psychometric properties of an assessment tool. To engage with this fully is beyond the scope of this chapter, but some of the key concepts are introduced next.

Validity

A valid measure will measure what it says it will, e.g. pain, work disability, hand function (Laver-Fawcett 2007). This is determined in a number of different ways including:

- Face validity: the extent to which the items appear to capture the concept being assessed. This is often established by asking clients to comment on the questions and whether any are not necessary or are missing and is therefore a subjective assessment.

- Criterion validity: the extent to which a measure correlates with another 'gold' standard measure which captures the same concept being measured, e.g. the extent to which a new measure of pain correlates with the McGill Pain Questionnaire. The new measure and 'gold' standard are administered at the same time and the level of correlation reported.
- Construct validity: the extent which an assessment tests an hypothesis related to what it is measuring, i.e. can it discriminate between people with early and late disease.

Reliability

Reliability refers to the ability of an assessment to produce consistent responses over time and between assessors (Laver-Fawcett 2007). There are a number of ways in which this is determined including:

- Internal consistency: the extent to which items measure the same underlying construct, e.g. pain or anxiety.
- Test–retest reliability: explores how stable an assessment is determined by asking the same people to complete the assessment on two occasions. For people who report no change in their condition between assessments, the two scores should be similar.
- Inter/intra-rater reliability: If an assessment involves observation or measurement of, e.g., range of movement, it is important to consider how reproducible the measurement is and how much measurement error may be present. This is established in two ways by either asking the same therapist to measure the same person on two different occasions (intra-rater reliability) or by asking different therapists to measure the same person (inter-rater reliability) and comparing the two measurements.

Responsiveness to change

This refers to the degree to which an assessment can pick up change and is reported in two ways:

- Sensitivity: refers to an assessments ability to detect change when change has occurred and is explored in the context of delivering an intervention.
- Minimum clinically important difference: provides an indication of what is a clinically important change in score as opposed to a statistically important change. For example, using the FIQ, a change in the total FIQ score of 8.1 represents a clinically meaningful change. This sets a benchmark against which to measure interventions (Bennet et al. 2009).

Is the assessment culturally relevant?

If working with people from different cultural backgrounds, the cultural relevance and language used in an assessment should be considered. Some of the more frequently used questionnaires have undergone cross-cultural validation, which means that a structured formal process has been followed to ensure that the items in the assessment are culturally relevant, that the translation is accurate and that the psychometric properties of the original questionnaire are replicated in the translated version. Evidence of this process should be available, and if it is not a 'translated' assessment should be used with caution as data derived may not be reliable and valid.

Other considerations

Copyright

Many standardised assessments are covered by copyright. This means that permission must be obtained from the author before it can be used and in some instances, e.g. the SF36 (Ware and Sherbourne 1992) or the Hospital Anxiety and Depression score (Zigmond and Snaith 1983), a charge is made for its use.

Ease of completion

Self-complete questionnaires rely on a fairly good level of literacy skills, and some people may experience difficulty and require some help or support.

Ease of scoring

The way in which questionnaires are scored varies considerably. Some require the scores to be summed to provide a total score, whilst others require a greater degree of interpretation and time to score.

Outcome Measures in Rheumatology

Outcome Measures in Rheumatology (OMERACT) is an international informal network founded to improve outcome measures in rheumatology (Tugwell et al. 2007). Focusing on specific areas of practice, a consensus-building approach is utilised to identify a core set of outcomes endorsed by OMERACT. To achieve OMERACT endorsement, an outcome has to pass the OMERACT filter (Table 5.10).

Over recent years clients have been increasingly involved in the OMERACT conferences and contributed to the consensus-building process. Details of the OMERACT proceedings can be found on their website www.intermed.med.uottawa.ca/research/omeract./publications/publicationsgeneral.html

Table 5.10 OMERACT filter.

Truth	Does the measure measure what it is meant to and is the result relevant and free from bias?
Discrimination	Does the measure have the ability to discriminate?
Feasibility	Is it feasible to use the measure in terms of cost, time and scoring?

5.6   Summary

A significant proportion of this chapter has been dedicated to the selection of appropriate assessments focusing specifically on the use of standardised assessments as one of the tools of data collection utilised in the assessment process. The integration of standardised assessments is central to the development and delivery of evidence-based practice and their use should be routine in the occupational therapy assessment process to meet both clinical and policy objectives.

Resources

Patient Outcomes in Rheumatology (2011) *Arthritis Care and Research* 63(S11). This is a special edition that provides one of the most comprehensive reviews of OMERACT practice covering over 250 measures.

The measurement of patient-reported outcome in the rheumatic diseases. Haywood K in Dziedzic K, Hammond A (eds.) (2010) *Rheumatology. Evidence-based Practice for Physiotherapists and Occupational Therapists*. New York: Churchill Livingstone.

References

Backman C, Mackie H, Harris J (1991) Arthritis hand function test: Development of a standardised tool. *Occupational Therapy Journal of Research* 11:246–256.

Bennett R, Bushmakin A, Cappelleri J, et al. (2009) Minimal clinically important difference in the Fibromyalgia Impact Questionnaire. *Journal of Rheumatology* 36:1304–1311.

Bowling A (2009) The psychometric properties of the Older People's Quality of Life Questionnaire, compared with the CASP-19 and the WHOQOL-OLD. *Current Gerontology and Geriatrics Research*. http://www.hindawi.com/journals/cggr/2009/298950/. Accessed on 29 March 2012.

Burckhardt R, Clark S, Bennett R (1991) The Fibromyalgia Impact Questionnaire: Development and validation. *Journal of Rheumatology* 18(5):728–733.

Carr A, Hewlett S, Hughes R, et al. (2003) Rheumatology outcomes: The patient's perspective. *The Journal of Rheumatology* 30(4):880–883.

College of Occupational Therapists (COT) (2003) *Occupational Therapy Clinical Guidelines for Rheumatology*. London: COT.

COT (2010) *Code of Ethics and Professional Conduct*. London: COT.

COT (2011) *Professional Standards for Occupational Therapy Practice*. London: COT.

Dawson J, Fitzpatrick R, Carr A, et al. (1996) Questionnaire on the perceptions of patients about total hip replacement. *Journal of Bone and Joint Surgery (Br)* 78(2):185–190.

Dawson J, Fitzpatrick R, Murray D, et al. (1998) Questionnaire on the perceptions of patients about total knee replacement. *Journal of Bone Joint Surgery (Br)* 80(1):63–69.

Department of Health (DoH) (2008) *Guidance on the Routine Collection of Patient Reported Outcome Measures*. London: DoH.

DoH (2009) *Guidance on the Routine Collection of Patient Reported Outcome Measures*. London: DoH. http://www.dh.gov.uk/en/Publicationsandstatistics/Publications/Publications PolicyAndGuidance/DH_092647. Accessed on 29 March 2012.

DoH (2010) *Equity and Excellence: Liberating the NHS*. London: DoH. http://www.dh.gov. uk/en/Publicationsandstatistics/Publications/PublicationsPolicyAndGuidance/ DH_117353. Accessed on 29 March 2012.

EuroQol Group (1990) EuroQol – A new facility for the measurement of health-related quality of life. *Health Policy* 16(3):199–208.

Fox M, Martin P, Green G (2007) *Doing Practitioner Research*. London: Sage.

Fries J, Spitz P, Young D (1982) The dimensions of outcomes: The Health Assessment Questionnaire, disability and pain scales. *Arthritis and Rheumatism* 9:789–793.

Garratt A, Schmidt L, Mackintosh A, et al. (2002) Quality of life measurement: Bibliographic study of patient assessed health outcome measures. *British Medical Journal* 324:1417.10.

Gilworth G, Chamberlain M, Harvey A, et al. (2003) Development of a work instability scale for rheumatoid arthritis. *Arthritis Rheumatism* 49:349–354.

Goodacre L, Smith J, Meddis D, et al. (2007) Development and validation of a measure of activity limitation. *Rheumatology* 46:703–708.

Greenhalgh T, Hurwitz B (1999) 'Why study narrative?' *British Medical Journal* 318:48–50.

Hammond A (1996) Functional and health assessments used in rheumatology occupational therapy: A review and United Kingdom survey. *British Journal of Occupational Therapy* 59(6):254–259.

Haywood K, Garratt A, Jordan K, et al. (2010) Evaluation of Ankylosing Spondylitis Quality of Life (EASi-QoL): Reliability and validity of a new patient-reported outcome measure. *The Journal of Rheumatology* 37(10):2100–2109.

Hewlett S (2003) Patients and clinicians have different perspectives of outcomes in arthritis. *Journal of Rheumatology* 30(4):877–879.

Hewlett S, Smith A, Kirwan J (2001) Values for function in rheumatoid arthritis. Patients, professionals and public. *Annals of Rheumatic Diseases* 60:928–933.

Laver-Fawcett A (2007) *Principles of Assessment and Outcome for Occupational Therapists and Physiotherapists. Theory, Skills and Application*. Chichester, UK: John Wiley & Sons, Ltd.

Law M, Baptiste S, McColl M, et al. (1990) The Canadian occupational performance measure: An outcome measure for occupational therapy. *Canadian Journal of Occupational Therapy* 57(2):82–87.

Lorig K, Brown B, Ung E, et al. (1989) Development and evaluation of a scale to measure the perceived self-efficacy of people with arthritis. *Arthritis and Rheumatism* 32(1):37–44.

Macedo A, Oakley S, Panayi G, et al. (2009) Functional outcomes improve in patient with rheumatoid arthritis who receive targeted, comprehensive occupational therapy. *Arthritis and Rheumatism* 61(11):1522–1530.

Meenan R, Mason J, Anderson J, et al. (1992) AIMS2: The content and properties of a revised and expanded Arthritis Impact Measurement Scales Health Status Questionnaire. *Arthritis and Rheumatism* 35(1):1–10.

Melzack R (1975) The McGill Pain Questionnaire: Major properties and scoring methods. *Pain* 1:277–299.

Melzack R (1987) The short-form McGill Pain Questionnaire. *Pain* 30:191–197.

Myers H, Thomas E, Hay E, et al. (2011) Hand assessment in older adults with musculoskel- etal hand problems: A reliability study. *BMC Musculoskeletal Disorder* 12:3. http://www. biomedcentral.com/1471-2474/1/2/3. Accessed on 29 March 2012.

NHS Scotland (2010) *NHS Scotland Quality Strategy. Putting People at the Heart of the NHS*. http://www.scotland.gov.uk/Publications/2010/05/10102307/0. Accessed on 29 March 2012.

Prevoo L, Van't Hof M, Kuper H, et al. (1995) Modified disease activity scores that include twenty-eight–joint counts: Development and validation in a prospective longitudinal study of patients with rheumatoid arthritis. *Arthritis Rheumatism* 38:44–48.

Spitzer R, Kroenke K, Williams J (1999) Validation and utility of a self-report versions of PRIME-MD: The PHQ Primary Care Study. *Journal of the American Medical Association* 282:1737–1744.

Stein M, Wallston K, Nicassio P (1988) Factor structure of the Arthritis Helplessness Index. *Journal of Rheumatology* 15:427–432.

Tugwell P, Boers M, Brooks P, et al. (2007) OMERACT: An international initiative to improve outcome measurement in rheumatology. *Trials* 8:38.

Van Lankveld W, Van't Pad Bosch P, Bakker J, et al. (1996) Sequential Occupational Dexterity Assessment (SODA): A new test to measure hand disability. *Journal of Hand Therapy* 9:27–32.

Ware J, Sherbourne C (1992) The MOS 36-item Short-form Health Survey (SF36). Conceptual framework and item selection. *Medical Care* 30:473–483.

Ware J, Kosinski M, Keller S (1996) A 12-item Short-Form Health Survey: Construction of scales and preliminary tests of reliability and validity. *Medical Care* 34:220 233.

Ware J, Kosinski M, Dewey J, et al. (2001) How to score and interpret single-item health status measures: *A manual for users of the SF-8 Health Survey*. Lincoln, RI: QualityMetric Incorporated.

Welsh Government (2011) *Together for Health. A 5 Year Vision for the NHS in Wales*. http:// new.wales.gov.uk/topics/health/publications/health/reports/together/?lang=en. Accessed on 29 March 2012.

Zigmond A, Snaith R (1983) The hospital anxiety and depression scale. *Acta Psychiatrica Scandinavica* 67:361–370.

Chapter 6

Psychological approaches to understanding and managing rheumatic conditions

Deborah Harrison

School of Allied Health Professions, University of East Anglia, Norfolk, United Kingdom

6.1 Introduction

This chapter will connect theories and approaches from health psychology with occupational therapy practice in order to support the clinical reasoning of occupational therapists working with people who have rheumatic conditions. Health psychology will be defined and the biopsychosocial model discussed to establish the shared understanding that health psychologists and occupational therapists have about the key role that psychological and social processes play in the experience of living with a rheumatic condition. Psychological theories relevant to living with long-term illness will be described and illustrated with client narratives. The implications for occupational therapy practice will be explored.

6.2 Health psychology and biopsychosocial perspectives

Health psychology applies psychological theories to understanding the experience of health and illness (Morrison and Bennett 2009). The main goals of health psychology are:

- Promoting and maintaining health
- Improving health care and systems and health policy
- Preventing and treating illness
- Understanding the causes of illness, for example, vulnerability/risk factors

With these goals in mind, occupational therapists study psychology in their pre-registration programmes and understand the important foundations that psychological

Rheumatology Practice in Occupational Therapy: Promoting Lifestyle Management, First Edition.
Edited by Lynne Goodacre and Margaret McArthur.
© 2013 John Wiley & Sons, Ltd. Published 2013 by John Wiley & Sons, Ltd.

theories provide to their practice in health and social care. As clinicians, occupational therapists are therefore familiar with the insights provided by psychology into a wide variety of topics like learning, motivation, personality and emotion, and they know that these all have relevance when trying to understand health and illness (Morrison and Bennett 2009). Health psychology, like occupational therapy, poses a challenge to the biomedical model (Ogden 2007) by offering an understanding that the causes and experiences of illness go beyond the purely biological or physical and encompass also psychological and social factors.

The biopsychosocial model (Engel 1977) provides an important theoretical underpinning for health psychology (Morrison and Bennett 2009) and for occupational therapy. The understanding that physical health is influenced by psychological and social factors has become well established and is supported by research evidence. MacKinnon and Luecken (2008) state that as health psychology has matured, it has moved beyond establishing major relationships between just two variables, like pain and emotion for example, to exploring more complex relationships between a number of variables. Research questions now explore individual differences in the relationships between biological, psychological and social factors. Each person will be influenced to a different degree by differing issues. This recognises what occupational therapists have always understood through their clinical reasoning, that in the provision of therapy 'one size does not fit all' (MacKinnon and Luecken 2008, p. 1). Treatment plans have to be tailored to the individual goals of each client.

People with rheumatological conditions will be coping with complex challenges like pain and fatigue, which cannot be analysed with simple cause and effect relationships, even if they take into account psychological issues. Levels of fatigue will be influenced by a number of different factors, for example, physiological and neurological aspects of the condition, stress levels, emotional reactions, past experience, knowledge and understanding of the condition, expectations about the condition and reactions from the immediate social group. These different elements will be weighted in different ways for each individual in terms of how much they influence the experience of fatigue and then how the person reacts to their symptoms. For one person, the social environment may have a huge impact at a particular point in time, for another it might be their emotional reactions.

This understanding translates clinically into the delivery of health care, is informed by the biopsychosocial model, and acknowledges that there will be an individual response to every condition and treatment outcomes. This individual response will be heavily influenced by the person's understanding of their situation and their emotional reaction to it, and their behaviour will be affected as a result (Ogden 2007).

The concept of working holistically is therefore embedded in the philosophy of the biopsychosocial model and is well recognised by occupational therapists as a useful framework to inform their clinical reasoning. Macedo et al. (2009) found that a comprehensive occupational therapy intervention based on the biopsychosocial model significantly improved functional outcomes for people with rheumatoid arthritis at risk of losing their job. Although occupational therapists give full consideration to the psychological and social factors in the lived experience of rheumatic condition in their clinical reasoning, within time constraints and workload pressures it might not be possible to reflect this fully in the planning and delivery of therapy. Gettings (2010) found from a review of the literature that the treatment most commonly offered to people with rheumatoid arthritis by the multidisciplinary team did not focus on their psychological needs. This review states that the psychological welfare of people with rheumatoid arthritis is an important issue because the condition is strongly associated with anxiety, depression and low self-esteem (Gettings 2010), highlighting the importance of addressing the psychological impact of long-term, progressive and disabling rheumatological conditions alongside the treatment of the physical symptoms. This chapter will now describe some of the health psychology theories relevant to supporting clinical reasoning and understanding their influences on how a person might respond to and cope with the condition and therapy. Theoretical connections with occupational therapy will be discussed with the implications for interventions.

6.3 Coping with illness

A number of health psychology theories like Moos and Shafer's Crisis Theory and Leventhal's self-regulatory model of illness cognitions (Ogden 2007) state that an individual faced with a stressor, like illness, will actively seek to understand their situation. People do not respond passively to frightening events. For example, an individual who experiences new and painful symptoms will immediately start trying to make sense of what is happening to them, a cognitive process called appraisal.

6.4 Transactional model of stress

The perception or appraisal of an event as being a threat is an important component of whether that event is experienced as stressful. The transactional model of stress developed by Lazarus and Folkman (1987, cited in Ogden 2007) identifies an active process of interaction with the event and undertaking a primary and secondary appraisal of the potential stress. Primary appraisal involves deciding whether there is actually a threat in terms of harm already done, a future threat of harm or a challenge that might pose an opportunity. Secondary appraisal involves a decision about the resources available to deal with the threat posed, and the stress can be reduced by a positive secondary appraisal (Morrison and Bennett 2009).

These two interacting processes are governed by *influencing factors* which include age, gender, temporal issues, values and beliefs, information skills, physiological arousal, empowerment, social support, efficacy, novelty and mood (Gage 1992). Elements of primary and secondary appraisal are examined, informed by the influencing factors and brought together into a *coping plan* which is evaluated through *outcome appraisal*. The efficacy and desirability of that outcome are re-appraised by reviewing the primary and secondary appraisals of the situation and also through reflecting on the influencing factors. If after re-appraisal the outcome seems to be a reasonable solution to the problem, the *final outcome* is acknowledged. If the solution is somehow seen as unacceptable, the whole process may begin again (Figure 6.1).

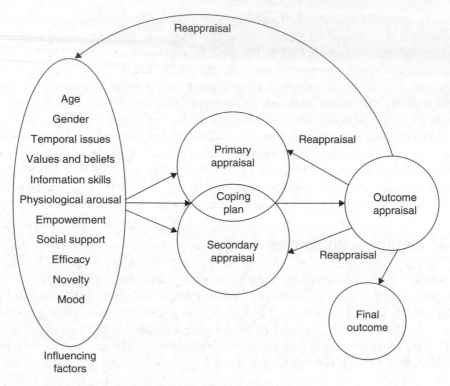

Figure 6.1   Diagrammatic representation of appraisal processes.

All of the influencing factors inform the primary and secondary appraisal activities (Gage 1992). An example of appraisal is when Anne was asked to talk about how she first developed rheumatoid arthritis. She presented the events in the form of a narrative. The narrative could be viewed as an appraisal of her search for an explanation for her symptoms. While the narrative presents to account in chronological order, Anne moves through all the stages of appraisal in a cyclical rather than a linear process (Figure 6.2).

It is possible that the process would only begin again if the influencing factors were strong enough to allow people to feel that they can do something about the problem. These perceptions are important to address if therapists are going to effectively work with this client group.

Occupational therapists can use their understanding of the role of appraisal in stress to explore a person's expectations and understanding about their rheumatic conditions during assessment, particularly when a person is first diagnosed. The provision of clear and honest information about the condition is essential to help a person feel that they have the resources to face the challenges posed by the condition and they may then be more likely to, for example, adhere to joint protection strategies as a result. On the other hand, if they have a negative view of the condition being untreatable and their ability to cope with it as fragile, they might feel overwhelmed and feel that adhering to therapy

Narrative	Appraisal Phase
I used to get fluid on my knees when I was a teenager	**Influencing factors** *physiological arousal; age; information skills*
I do kneeling at work and you don't know whether you've twisted your knees or anything do you	**Primary appraisal**
I said to my mum, 'There is something wrong there'	**Secondary appraisal**
I mean I was in agony but I kept putting cream on it to help it	**Coping plan**
but it weren't really helping	**Outcome appraisal**
I am a person I cannot sit down, that's my problem	**Influencing factors** *values and beliefs; temporal issues; physiological arousal*
This (*rheumatoid arthritis*), you got to keep resting, you can't sort of keep going all the time like you normally would	**Secondary appraisal**
I said, 'I don't know I think we'll get the doctor out and see what it is'	**Primary appraisal** **Coping plan**
but when he came he didn't know what it was	**Outcome appraisal**
I think he thought I was mucking about to be honest	**Influencing factors** – *values and beliefs; empowerment*
I am a person who don't go to the doctors…I'll hang on and hang on as long as I can…I can't stand being ill, that drives me crackers	**Influencing factors** – *values and beliefs; temporal; efficacy; physiological arousal; mood*
He came back a week later and saw me and that was just as bad again. He said, 'I don't know but we had better start doing some blood tests'	**Outcome appraisal**
and then they found it (*she was diagnosed with RA*)	**Final outcome**

Figure 6.2   Example of primary and secondary appraisal activities (McArthur 2002).

is pointless. Occupational therapists, in promoting stress management strategies, can bring their understanding of appraisal processes into clinical reasoning by dedicating time to exploring people's beliefs and expectations about their condition.

6.5   Self-efficacy and hardiness

The concept of self-efficacy can be used to underpin their clinical reasoning when incorporating self-management programmes into occupational therapy practice. When an individual makes an appraisal of their ability to respond to a stressful event, as described earlier, it is strongly influenced by their self-efficacy. Self-efficacy refers to the amount of confidence a person has in their ability to cope and is related to how much control they feel they have over their situation, also described as mastery. This narrative from Ruth illustrates self-efficacy, 'I'm that kind of person...I like to know the different alternative treatments and I like to know what to expect if things go wrong...I was straight round the library gathering the books...'. This confidence and feeling of control is enhanced when treatment approaches, like self-management, which seek to increase a person's self-efficacy, are used. A systematic review of the literature into coping strategies and self-efficacy in osteoarthritis (Benyon et al. 2010) found that self-efficacy played a role in predicting levels of disability, although they did not find a connection between self-efficacy and pain. The authors argue that a better understanding of coping and self-efficacy would help clinicians and clients to manage the condition more effectively. Occupational therapy research into self-efficacy with clients who have scleroderma found that low levels of self-efficacy were related to depression, pain, fatigue and disability (Buck et al. 2010). The authors conclude that self-management programmes that address these issues can improve self-efficacy and, by implication, support the process of coping with a chronic illness (Buck et al. 2010).

Self-efficacy appears to be related to a trait that some people possess called hardiness. People who are hardy have a strong sense of control over their lives, as well as the confidence and commitment to face challenges (Ogden 2007). The concept of hardiness was developed some time ago (Kobasa 1979, cited in Morrison and Bennett 2009) but still has relevance in clinical reasoning today. The client-centred approach used by occupational therapists means that they will be aware of these factors and will plan therapy to exploit the strengths of the individual. Collaborative goal setting and self-report devices like diaries support clients' feelings of being in control. Also, as we shall see in the following discussion, not all clients will come to therapy with a strong sense of having control over their situation.

6.6   Locus of control

There are individual differences in the ways that clients cope with a rheumatic condition, and not all clients will engage with therapy feeling confident and in control. The concept of locus of control is used to explain some of these individual differences in the way that people engage with behaviours that would promote their health and prevent disease. The theory, first proposed by Rotter (1966), was developed further by Wallston and Wallston (1982, cited in Ogden 2011). People with an internal locus of control consider themselves in control of their health and able to influence outcomes. This is similar to self-efficacy. A person with an external locus of control, however, believes that external forces are the prime determinates of health outcomes, rather than their own behaviour (Morrison and Bennett 2009), and individuals may feel their rheumatic condition is in control of their life and that they cannot do anything to improve their own health. Carol illustrates this sense of fate when she explained that 'I could remember my Auntie as an old lady with arthritis and hands that were all knobbly and everything and I thought that was how I was going to be – knobbly little old, not be able to get around…quite devastating really.'

An example of someone else who displayed an external locus of control was Anne who cited a number of difficult circumstances as proof that she is not in control (McArthur 2002). She recounted how:

- her father had died,
- her mother had been diagnosed as diabetic and had temporarily lost her eyesight,
- her daughter's car had been stolen,
- her daughter also had a number of personal problems,
- she had a number of serious health problems other than rheumatoid arthritis and
- a close family member had been involved in a car accident

all since she moved into her present house. She added that her neighbour had suffered some misfortune and concluded that their houses must be jinxed in some way, what she called a 'tizzy'. When she was asked if she really believed in fate, that she wasn't in control, she emphatically replied 'Yes…I always say to her (*her mother*) there must be a tizzy on this house'.

In addition to beliefs about fate, Kerns and Rosernburg (2000) also found individuals who held strong beliefs that their condition was purely physiological requiring medical attention would not engage in treatment approaches that emphasised personal responsibility, behaviour change or self-management.

Occupational therapists recognise that individuals adapt to their rheumatic condition in different ways based on how in control they feel, and for the client with an external locus of control it is necessary to factor this into the clinical reasoning. Occupational therapists can empower individuals to gain a greater internal locus of control through the establishment of effective therapeutic relationships, client-centred work and the provision of appropriate timely information. Therefore, where possible in rheumatology practice, occupational therapists involve the clients in the planning and implementation of interventions to promote their internal locus of control (McArthur 2002). Building treatment goals in small steps can quickly give a sense of success and progress. This is important because when clients have or develop an internal locus of control, they have the belief that their actions can impact on their health and treatment outcomes. These individuals are more self-motivated and likely to work alongside occupational therapists to make any necessary behaviour changes that they can to improve their health (McPherson et al. 2001). This moves the client towards a feeling that they are gaining control and can influence events, making a difference in effectively managing their own condition.

6.7 Crisis theory

Moos and Shaefer (1984, cited in Ogden 2007) provide a detailed theory within which to further frame understanding about the experience of coping with illness. They describe physical illness as a crisis, suggesting that people actively engage in a process of trying to reduce the impact of this on their lives. Crisis Theory describes five changes that an illness can bring, each of which has resonance with occupational therapy.

1 *Changes in identity*: Illness can result in a shift of identity. This is a change in the way that the person defines themselves or is seen by others. For example, a person may become a client or they might be conceived as a person with an illness or a disability. As a result, they might feel less of a person. Occupational therapists use a related term, occupational identity, which develops out of the occupations with which a person engages (Christian and Townsend 2004). The changes in occupations that arise from living with a rheumatic condition impact therefore on a person's identity. Engaging with the medical profession and therapists, for example, means that the person may define themselves in a traditional client role. This can be difficult because the change may feel like a loss of independence and control.

2 *Changes in location*: Illness may result in the person having to change location into hospital or becoming more confined to home. These changes may result in fewer opportunities to engage with everyday occupations, and occupational adaptation is necessary to cope with these limitations. As previously discussed, there is likely to be a feeling of losing control which could lower mood and motivation. Within a home setting, occupational therapists will be working with clients to adapt their occupations to changing circumstances. The provision of equipment or adaptations can also limit the extent of the restrictions that might result from reduced mobility or fatigue.

3 *Changes in role*: Moos and Shaefer identify that a person may have changed roles as a result of a long-term condition, defining it as moving from independence to being passive and dependent. This links closely with the changes in identity discussed earlier and the actual or perceived limitations that being a client or a disabled person can bring. As with the change in identity, this can result in a feeling of loss and depression. Del Fabro Smith et al. (2012) found that activities related to motherhood were severely affected by arthritis but they also found that a strong occupational identity was maintained by being resourceful and that holding on to being and doing as a mother was important. The changes in role and identity need not be negative if clients can be supported to participate in the occupations that are meaningful to them and help them to fulfil important roles.

4 *Changes in social support*: Illness can result in isolation from friends and family for a variety of reasons and this will have a negative impact on coping. A common experience for people with rheumatic conditions associated with high degrees of fatigue is one of being too tired to go out in the evenings, or if a person is in employment needing to spend the weekend resting and regaining energy for the week ahead. There might also be a hesitation from friends or family to keep in contact if they feel that they might overly fatigue the person for example. Or they might be embarrassed that they don't know what to say, or how to give support.

Loneliness will increase the negative impact of the other changes, particularly identity and role. This will lower feelings of self-efficacy and possibly result in depression and deterioration in the physical condition. Occupational therapists, in facilitating engagement in meaningful occupations, can address these issues with their clients. The concept of change in social support can be developed further than immediate friends and family. Occupational therapists will be aware of the broader, societal impacts of changes that result from the crisis of physical illness. People with a chronic condition resulting in disability can experience occupational deprivation from negative attitudes and discrimination in society (Christian and Townsend 2004; Harrison and Sellers 2008). Occupational therapists also act as advocates for their clients and are involved in developing Government policies to address inequalities.

5 *Changes in future*: The future becomes uncertain with the diagnosis of long-term illness, and this is one of the most difficult things to adjust to. The future will be different and there will be a need to readjust plans and acknowledge the loss that this might bring. With rheumatological conditions, plans for having children, travelling or work might be potentially threatened. For example, the negative impact of a rheumatic condition on continuing at work has been explored by occupational therapists (Macedo et al. 2010). As we shall see at the end of the chapter, a changed future does not need to mean that the future is bleak.

The model then states that the person engages in seven adaptive tasks: three illness-related tasks and four general tasks. The illness-related tasks arise as a result of having the condition:

1 Dealing with pain and symptoms of the illness
2 Dealing with the hospital environment and treatment
3 Developing and maintaining relationships with health professionals

These might be new tasks for the person at the beginning of their illness journey. They might have had little contact with the medical profession until their symptoms get so severe that they cannot avoid it. The narrative from a woman experiencing pain and limitation of movement in her knees illustrates this, 'I am a person who don't go to the doctors…I'll just hang on and hang on as long as I can…I can't stand being ill, that drives me crackers'.

Occupational therapists have a key role in supporting the coping mechanisms around the illness-related tasks, and building a positive therapeutic relationship is an important part of supporting the coping mechanisms around the illness-related tasks. Working as a part of the interprofessional team is essential to ensure that treatment and therapy are co-ordinated well.

The four general tasks are not specifically related to the illness and might be engaged with when undergoing any kind of stress or life change:

1 Preserving a reasonable emotional balance
2 Preserving a satisfactory self-image
3 Sustaining relationships
4 Preparing for an uncertain future

These tasks are connected with the changes in identity, social support and future discussed earlier. Successful engagement with these tasks facilitates coping and adjustment to the condition. By facilitating engagement in meaningful occupations, occupational therapists are well placed to support the individual to maintain a sense of identity, to feel competent and achieve mastery in their everyday life. It is through adapted occupations that the new future can be forged.

The third part of the coping process indentified by Moos and Shafer (1984, cited in Ogden 2007) are the coping skills, appraisal-focused, problem-focused and emotion-focused. These will be discussed in the next section.

6.8   Coping styles

Coping describes anything that a person does to reduce their experience of stress; it might not make the stressor go away, but it might reduce the impact that it has (Morrison and Bennett 2009). This process of adaptation is relevant for an individual living with a rheumatic condition because of all the changes and adaptations discussed previously. A number of different coping styles and two broad dimensions have been identified. An individual's coping style can be characterised as being problem-focused, emotion-focused, approach-focused or avoidant (Morrison and Bennett 2009).

- *Problem-focused coping* involves engaging actively in reducing the stressor or increasing the resources to deal with it. The person will seek practical support to address problems directly that arise from the situation.
- *Emotion-focused coping* involves dealing with the emotional responses to the stressor and might involve seeking support to see things in a more positive light or venting anger.
- *Approach-focused coping* is tackling the stressor directly by taking steps to reduce its effect, for example, by proactively searching for information about the condition.
- *Avoidant coping* is concerned with avoiding the stressor or minimising its threat and might involve avoiding situations or withdrawing by engaging in other activities or substance abuse.

Occupational therapists' awareness of the different coping styles that might be adopted by their clients enables them to support people in the most appropriate way. Although it might be intuitive to conclude that problem-focused and approach-focused coping are likely to be more adaptive, there is evidence that it is very dependent on the circumstances (Morrison and Bennett 2009). So, it is important to remember that, whatever the style of coping, it might be helping that person at that point in time (Ogden 2007), and the therapist must be non-judgemental about what they think is the 'correct' way to manage the condition. This analysis of coping styles can be helpful when reflecting on more challenging clients who, for example, may appear to be avoiding facing up to their situation. Understanding these individual differences in coping will support the clinical reasoning to adopt different communication styles. For example, it has been demonstrated that for preoperative preparation, people with an avoidant coping style might benefit from having less information whereas those with a problem-focused style appreciated having more (Morrison and Bennett 2009).

6.9   Moving beyond coping: hope

In mental health practice, the concept of recovery has become an important guide to the way that people can think about living with a long-term condition. A central component of the meaning of the word 'recovery' is hope; this does not refer to hope of a cure, but being able to forge a positive and meaningful life with the condition (COT 2006; Shepherd et al. 2008). A new field within psychology, referred to as 'positive psychology' (Morrison and Bennett 2009), also develops the theme of hope and suggests that we recognise the benefits of thinking and acting positively for health and well-being. Seligman (2003) introduced these ideas, and they have a strong resonance for occupational therapists. Happiness and joy are a part of a good life and this arises from not just being, but also doing. This means being involved with life and all of its activities. The simple pleasures that we can get out of life, particularly doing things for or with others, can make life meaningful and fulfilled. In a small study, Hawtin and Sullivan (2011) found indications that mindfulness training had the potential to improve the ability to cope with pain and psychological well-being for clients with rheumatological conditions. This positive and hopeful approach to life from psychological theory sits well with the philosophy of occupational therapy. In recognising that occupation is fundamental to human life (Yerxa 2000) and that it also has the power to transform lives when people have experienced ill-health or injury (Christiansen and Townsend 2004).

6.10   Conclusion

Occupational therapists combine knowledge of the psychological processes involved in coping with their occupational perspectives during their clinical reasoning. The result is a unique and holistic therapy that supports the person living with a rheumatic condition in both the physical, psychological and social challenges that they face. There is clear evidence and a strong argument to support occupational therapists continuing to address psychological and social needs with people living with rheumatic conditions even when services and resources are under pressure. Combining concepts and theories from occupational therapy with those from health psychology enhances the range of information contributing to good clinical reasoning. Awareness of individual differences and the complexity of factors influencing outcomes enhances the delivery of effective occupational therapy. Engagement in meaningful occupations promotes hope, health and well-being.

Resources

Advice on Self-Management. http://www.arthritiscare.org.uk/PublicationsandResources/Self management. Accessed on 14 November 2012.

Brief Information on Self-Management of Lupus. http://www.lupusuk.org.uk/managing-lupus. Accessed on 14 November 2012.

General Advice for Everyone on Promoting Mental Health Well-Being. http://www.nhs.uk/ LiveWell/mental-wellbeing/Pages/mental-wellbeing.aspx. Accessed on 14 November 2012.

Generic Advice on Self-Management of Long-Term Conditions for GPs. http://www.bma.org. uk/patients_public/selfmanagementresource.jsp. Accessed on 14 November 2012.

NICE Guideline for Rheumatoid Arthritis. http://guidance.nice.org.uk/CG79/Guidance/pdf/ English. Accessed on 14 November 2012.

Scottish Guidance on Promoting Mental Health and Well-Being for People with Long-Term Conditions. http://www.scotland.gov.uk/Publications/2009/06/02153313/3. Accessed on 14 November 2012.

References

Benyon K, Hill S, Zadurian N, et al. (2010) Coping strategies and self-efficacy as predictors of outcomes in osteoarthritis: A systematic review. *Musculoskeletal Care* 8:224–236.

Buck U, Poole J, Mendelson C (2010) Factors relating to self-efficacy in persons with scleroderma. *Musculoskeletal Care* 8:197–203.

Christiansen CH, Townsend EA (2004) *Introduction to Occupation: The Art and Science of Living*. Upper Saddle River, NJ: Prentice Hall.

College of Occupational Therapists (COT) (2006) *Recovering Ordinary Lives: The Strategy for Occupational Therapy in Mental Health Services, the Next Ten Years (Core)*. London: COT.

Del Fabro Smith L, Suto M, Chalmers A, et al. (2012) Belief in doing and knowledge in being mothers with arthritis. *Occupational Therapy Journal of Research: Occupation, Participation and Health* 31(1):40–48.

Engel GL (1977) The need for a new medical model: A challenge for biomedicine. *Science* 196:129–136.

Gettings L (2010) Psychological well-being in rheumatoid arthritis: A review of the literature. *Musculoskeletal Care* 8:99–106.

Harrison D, Sellers A (2008) Occupation for mental health and social inclusion. *British Journal of Occupational Therapy* 71(5):216–219.

Hawtin H, Sullivan C (2011) Experiences of mindfulness training in living with rheumatic condition: An interpretative phenomenological analysis. *British Journal of Occupational Therapy* 74(3):137–142.

Macedo AM, Oakley SP, Panayi GS, et al. (2009) Functional and work outcomes to improve in patients with rheumatoid arthritis who receive targeted and comprehensive occupational therapy. *Arthritis and Rheumatism* 61(11):1522–1530.

MacKinnon DP, Luecken LJ (2008) How and for whom? Mediation and moderation in health psychology. *Health Psychology* 27(2 Suppl):S99–100.

McArthur MA (2002) *Unheard Stories, Unmet Needs: The Clinical and Educational Implications of Perceptions of Rheumatoid Arthritis*. Norfolk, UK: Centre for Applied Research in Education, School of Education and Professional Development, University of East Anglia.

Morrison V, Bennett P (2009) *An Introduction to Health Psychology* (2nd edn.). Harlow, UK: Pearson Education Ltd.

Ogden J (2007) *Health Psychology: A Text Book* (4th edn.). Maidenhead, UK: Open University Press.

Seligman MEP (2003) Positive psychology: Fundamental assumptions. *The Psychologist* 16:126–127.

Shepherd G, Boardman J, Slade M (2008) *Making Recovery a Reality*. London: Sainsbury Centre for Mental Health.

Yerxa EJ (2000) Occupational science: A renaissance of service to humankind through knowledge. *Occupational Therapy International* 7(2):87–98.

Chapter 7

Approaches to promoting behaviour change

Sarah Drake

School of Allied Health Professions, University of East Anglia, Norfolk, United Kingdom

7.1 Introduction

This chapter considers 'health behaviour' and explores the key models around health behaviour change. It provides an overview of a number of different approaches to understanding health behaviour change and explores how these can be incorporated into therapeutic interventions by occupational therapists working with individuals with rheumatic conditions. The chapter then concludes by providing a worked example of the application of the Trans-Theoretical Model (TTM) to this area of practice. This model has been chosen to illustrate how models of health behaviour can be integrated into clinical practice to facilitate the process of behaviour change.

Health behaviours are behaviours related to the health and well-being of individuals and can be divided into two areas – health-impairing and health-protective habits:

Health-impairing habits (behavioural pathogens) are behaviours that can have a negative impact on health, for example smoking, a high-fat diet or consumption of large amounts of alcohol.

Health-protective habits (behavioural immunogens) are behaviours that may have a positive effect on health such as complying with medical advice, having regular checkups and having regular sleep and a good diet. In rheumatology practice, the health protective habit could be complying with joint protection advice (Matarazzo 1984, pp. 3–40, cited in Ogden 2011, p. 14).

Rheumatology Practice in Occupational Therapy: Promoting Lifestyle Management, First Edition.
Edited by Lynne Goodacre and Margaret McArthur.
© 2013 John Wiley & Sons, Ltd. Published 2013 by John Wiley & Sons, Ltd.

7.2   Relevance to occupational therapists

Helping individuals to change and adapt their health behaviours to promote health and well-being is important to the management of long-term conditions. This is especially relevant for people with rheumatic conditions as a strong emphasis on improving and adapting the functioning of individuals could work towards ameliorating long-term disability (Davis et al. 1994). As occupational therapists, many of our interventions require an element of behaviour change such as changing the way an everyday activity is carried out or adopting a new pattern of behaviour. It is this process of adaptation and development of new behaviours that necessitates the process of change (Dubouloz et al. 2008). Therefore, facilitating behaviour change is a key part of occupational therapy practice.

The process of change is complex and advising people to make changes and providing information around this is not enough to encourage an individual to change behaviour (Morrison and Bennett 2009). Understanding an individual's readiness to change, appreciating barriers to change and helping individuals anticipate potential areas of relapse of health impairing habits can improve overall client satisfaction and lower frustration during the change process (Zimmerman et al. 2007). Assessing an individual's readiness to change will enable treatment approaches to be adapted and tailored to facilitate this process of change.

Steultjens et al. (2004, cited in Dubouloz et al. 2008, p. 31) identified that occupational therapists work with clients with rheumatic conditions to enable them to modify their occupational performance. This could be through splinting, lifestyle management, joint protection advice or the use of assistive devices. These health behaviours are often not maintained due to individuals being resistant to change or lacking the belief that these changes will result in improvement. Therefore, to ensure the efficacy of service delivery, it is critical to understand the process of change, because if the process is misunderstood, occupational therapy interventions can be misdirected and less effective.

7.3   Health behaviour change

There are a number of theories and models that can be employed by occupational therapists to predict, explain and underpin interventions to promote behaviour change. Hillsdon et al. (2005, cited in Thirlaway and Upton 2009, p. 45) found that interventions based on these theories are associated with longer-term behaviour change in comparison to interventions with no theoretical underpinning. This reinforces the importance of incorporating behavioural change theory into practice.

The locus of control (LoC) theory was discussed in Chapter 6. This theory can be used to understand health behaviour change, as it highlights that individuals are more likely to change when they feel in control of their health. As well as the LoC theory, there are other theories that inform our understanding of behaviour change, and this chapter will focus on the theories of Unrealistic Optimism (UO) and Social Cognition (SC). Two models of exploring behaviour change, the Health Beliefs Model (HBM) and the TTM, will then be explored.

Unrealistic Optimism theory

This theory suggests that one of the reasons individuals engage in risky or unhealthy health behaviours is due to their inaccurate perceptions of risk. This could be their perception of the severity of their illness or their perception of their susceptibility to becoming ill in the first instance. Weinstein (1984) described four cognitive factors that contribute to UO:

1 Lack of personal experience with the problem
2 The belief that the illness is preventable by the individual
3 The belief that if a problem has not appeared it will never appear
4 The belief that the problem is infrequent and therefore is not a problem

Individuals focus on risk-reducing behaviours that they engage in and ignore risk-increasing behaviours. For example, an individual with a rheumatic condition may not adhere to the joint protection advice around problem solving, prioritising, planning and pacing during the day, but justify this risk-increasing behaviour by wearing a resting splint at night. The individual may believe that the splint is sufficient to prevent any biomechanical stress caused by not adhering to the joint protection advice and so not comprehend that their behaviour during the day could counteract any potential benefits of the splint. Providing client education can address this by increasing an individual's knowledge and understanding of their rheumatic condition. Taol et al. (1996) highlighted that client education can result in behaviour change, thus reinforcing the importance of consistently using joint protection techniques throughout the day and evening.

7.4 Social Cognition theories

SC theories including the Theory of Reasoned Action (TRA) and the Theory of Planned Behaviour (TPB) seek to understand clients' treatment decisions by focusing on the beliefs they hold about their illness (Goodacre and Goodacre 2004). SC theories look beyond the individuals as information processes and attempt to place the individual within the context of other people and the broader social world (Ogden 2011). It therefore considers the impact of other people and their views on the individual's decision to change/not change.

The Theories of Reasoned Action and Planned Behaviour

The TRA was first developed by Fishbein (1967, cited in Ogden 2011, p. 30) and explores the relationship between an individual's attitudes and behaviours within a social world (reasoned behaviour). According to the TRA, if individuals evaluate the suggested health behaviour as positive (attitude), and if they think their significant others want them to perform the health behaviour (subjective norm), this results in higher intention (motivation) increasing the likelihood of a health behaviour change (Maio and Haddock 2009).

TRA was developed into the TPB by Ajzen and Madden (1986, cited in Ogden 2011, p. 30). The TPB proposed that attitude towards behaviour, subjective norms and perceived behavioural control together shape an individual's behavioural intentions and behaviours. The development of this model from the TRA focused on perceived behavioural control, which explored the impact of confidence and control on an individual's intention to carry out particular health behaviours (Miller 2005). The TPB emphasised that behavioural intentions were an outcome of a combination of several beliefs:

- The individual's *attitude* towards particular health behaviours and the belief around the outcome of a behaviour change.
  A clinical example of this would be Beth, who believes that using a kettle tipper is beneficial for her joint protection but may feel it symbolises disability to others and clutters the kitchen. The theory suggests that Beth will only use the kettle tipper if she values the potential benefits of using it more than her other concerns.
- The *subjective norm* looks at the influence of other people's opinions on the individual's behavioural intentions.
  Beth may use the kettle tipper at home but when she tries to use one at work her work colleagues may make unhelpful comments about it or remove it from the work top. The opinions of these colleagues, weighted by the importance Beth attributes to each of those opinions, will influence her behavioural intention. If Beth values the benefits more than the opinion of her colleagues, she will continue to use the kettle tipper at work. However, if she places more value on colleagues' opinions, this will impact on her behavioural intention and she may stop using it, highlighting the influence external factors can have on an individual's behaviour.
- *Perceived behavioural control* focuses on individual's perceptions of whether they have the internal resources (skills, abilities, information) and external control factors (opportunities and obstacles) required to carry out a particular health behaviour. The concept of perceived behavioural control is conceptually related to self-efficacy (see Chapter 6).
  Thus, Beth has to feel confident that she can assert her views and continue to use the kettle tipper despite the comments and actions of her colleagues. If Beth feels that the colleagues' action (moving the kettle tipper) is an obstacle, this will impact on her intention to continue to use it.

7.5   Implications for practice

The TPB proposes that individuals only take action to change a health behaviour if they feel the change will benefit their overall health, if they are confident in their own belief and if they feel they have the internal resources to make the change happen. To facilitate behaviour change, occupational therapists could focus on increasing the individual's belief that there are benefits to changing and that the individual has the internal resources required to make the change.

Health Beliefs Model

The HBM was one of the first behaviour change models developed. It was initially developed by Rosenstock in 1966 but was developed further by Rosenstock and Becker (1974, cited in Morrison and Bennett 2009, pp. 131–136) to predict preventative health behaviours and the behavioural response to treatment in acutely and chronically ill people (Ogden 2011). The HBM proposes that the likelihood that a person will engage in particular health behaviours is a result of a set of core beliefs which the individual will have developed over a period of time. It suggests that individual belief in a personal threat together with belief in the effectiveness of adopting preventative (health) behaviour will predict the likelihood of that behaviour (Thirlaway and Upton 2009). The core beliefs are an individual's perception of:

- *Susceptibility* – 'my chances of getting ill are high/low'.
  Perceived threat from a disease strongly influences behavioural change (Hammond et al. 2004). If Individuals view their rheumatic condition as severe but feel they would be the same or better in 5 years time, this will result in a limited sense of susceptibility (Hammond et al. 1999).
- *Severity* – 'this illness is a trivial'.
  Dubouloz et al. (2008) highlighted that due to the fluctuating and invisible nature of rheumatic symptoms, individuals can develop hope for improvement and cure without them having to change their health behaviour; a remission phase can lead some individuals to hope that the condition is not severe or that they are cured.
- *Costs* – 'It will be easy/difficult to change my health behaviours – changing will result in...'.
  Hammond et al. (1999) identified that it is more likely that behaviour change would take place when an individual's perceived benefits and personal belief in their ability to change outweigh the perceived barriers.
- *Benefits* – 'I'll get a lot/little out of the change'.
  People have to feel they have something pertinent and significant to gain from making a change. If they identify limited or no benefits in considering self-management techniques, they are less likely to contemplate health behaviour changes (Hammond et al. 2004).
- *Cues to action – internal cues (symptoms) external trigger (such as a health education leaflet).*
  People with rheumatic conditions may not always have the physical experience of pain and fatigue. If they are in a period of remission, they may feel that things are more tolerable (Hammond et al. 2004). Reduction in the physical experience of pain for the individual can reduce the internal cue to action. Conversely, individuals can be prompted to change their health behaviours when they are experiencing uncomfortable symptoms or they have an emotional reaction to an external trigger.
- *Health motivation – readiness to be concerned about health and well-being.*
  Health motivation explores how ready an individual is to be concerned about their health. If individuals do not feel concerned about their current health behaviours

negatively affecting their condition, they will not be motivated to make any changes (Zimmerman 2007). When individuals believe that changing their health behaviours can impact on their health and potentially result in an improvement to their health, their health motivation increases (McPherson et al. 2001).

• *Perceived control* – 'I am confident that I can change/I've tried before and I can't do it'.

Kerns and Rosernburg (2000) and Taol et al. (1996) highlighted that self-efficacy strongly influences behavioural choices and decisions, and the unpredictable course and fluctuating disease activity in rheumatic conditions can contribute to feelings that the condition is uncontrollable, thus lowering the sense of self-efficacy. In the same way, if people feel their rheumatic condition can only be managed by medical interventions rather than through self-management, they will have an impaired sense of personal control over their health.

7.6 Implications for practice

The HBM proposes that individuals only take action to change if they value their health, perceive a threat to it and feel confident that they can successfully take actions that could eliminate or minimise the threat (Freeman et al. 2002). If individuals do not perceive a threat, they will not take action. Therefore, if individuals with rheumatic conditions are experiencing minimal biomechanical disruptions and moderate levels of pain and fatigue, they may not change or adapt their behaviours. To facilitate behaviour change, occupational therapists could explore an individual's perceived susceptibility, severity, barriers and benefits of change whilst also focusing on improving the individual's sense of self-efficacy. To facilitate behaviour change, the perceived benefits and belief in their own ability to change needs to outweigh the barriers to changing behaviour.

The Trans-Theoretical Model

The TTM initially focused on smoking cessation but is relevant to other areas of practice which target changes in health behaviours that are causing harm (Prochaska and Diclemente (1984, cited in DiClemente et al. 1991). It is pertinent to rheumatology practice because it highlights that clients with rheumatic conditions may be at different stages of change when adopting self-management strategies (Keefe et al. 2000).

The TTM resonates with/incorporates theories and models previously discussed including the HBM and the UO theory. The TTM explores the process of making a change in behaviour and proposes that individual's cycle through different stages of change, and the processes involved at the different stages vary (Morrison and Bennett 2009). People can move from one stage to another very quickly or remain in one of the stages for a long time. The movement from one stage to another is not necessarily cyclical and individuals may move back to earlier stages. If an individual relapses, this does not necessarily signify that they have gone right back to the beginning but that they may have just moved back to a previous stage which needs to be considered when planning interventions.

The TTM proposes that different cognitions are important at different stages and identifying an individual's position in the stages facilitates tailoring the intervention to match that stage (Diclemente and Hughes 1990). For example, in the earlier stages, information may be processed about the costs and benefits of changing behaviour, whilst in the later stages cognitions become more focused on the development of plans of action to initiate and support the maintenance of behaviour. Identifying the factors that promote progression and influence relapse between the stages of change is beneficial to facilitate progression.

7.7 Motivational interviewing

Motivational interviewing (MI) – a non-directive client-centred approach in which the interviewer facilitates the development of an individual's motivation.
Mindfulness – moment-to-moment non-judgemental attention and awareness actively cultivated and developed through meditation (Pradhan et al. (2007).

Miller and Rollnick (2002) highlighted that MI can be key in facilitating peoples' progression and that different processes of change can be applied at the different stages. MI is used in a wide range of health contexts including chronic disease management and can address a wide range of behaviours including negative lifestyle behaviours. It is particularly useful in the early stages of change to encourage individuals to express their ambivalence about behaviour change, to help identification of reasons for resistance towards change and to facilitate moving towards behaviour change at a measured pace. The approach encourages the individual to initiate the behaviour change and take responsibility for that change in contrast to the therapist arguing the case for change. Therefore, MI helps individuals to reach these decisions for themselves (Rollnick et al. 1992). It is versatile, and with support and training occupational therapists can use this approach to facilitate behaviour change and encourage individuals to move forward in the stages of change (Figure 7.1).

7.8 Clinical example of the TTM

Edward was in his early 50s and co-owned a 250 acre farm with his two brothers. He was diagnosed with rheumatoid arthritis one year ago. He was struggling with the more physically demanding tasks on the farm and was experiencing high levels of pain and fatigue. He was advised to make some changes to his work routine including

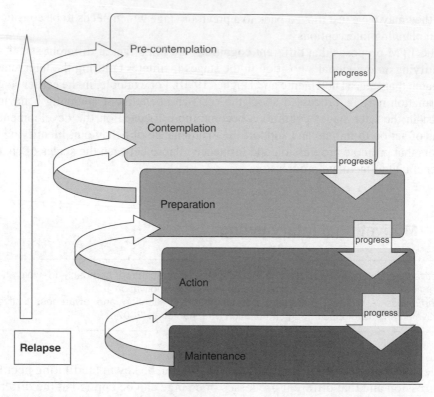

Figure 7.1 The Trans-Theoretical Model.

handing over the heavier tasks on the farm, including milking the cows, to his brothers to prevent aggravating his symptoms and to reduce the biomechanical disruption of his condition. Edward's process of adapting to this change in his work routine is demonstrated (Table 7.1).

Pre-contemplation

> I took the shed to pieces moved it all away and one morning I got up and all my hand was like that (swollen)…so whether there was something on the wood, I suppose you get little old mites and different things in it, well this thumb about 2.30 am I had to get out of bed and sit in the lounge because I couldn't do anything with my hands.

- Edward demonstrated an external LoC. He did not feel that the physical task of taking the shed down was to blame for the exacerbation of his symptoms.
- Edward was offered an alternative explanation for the pain in his thumb, but he reiterated that it was something on the wood that caused his increased pain. Therefore, he felt he had no control over the situation and no need to change his behaviour.

Table 7.1   The pre-contemplation stage of the TTM.

Stage of change	Characteristics
Pre-contemplation Not intending to make changes	Tend to be unaware of the need to change and maybe in denial about the seriousness of the condition therefore are resistant to modify their behaviour (Unrealistic Optimism)
	There are two types of pre-contemplators:
	Aware pre-contemplators – people who know they are maintaining unhelpful behaviours but do not intend to change
	Unaware pre-contemplators – people who do not perceive that they have unhelpful behaviours and therefore experience no need to change (Lechner et al. 1998, cited in Burg et al. 2005)

Processes of change to encourage health behaviour change

- *Consciousness raising* – provide small amounts of information to ensure the individual has an accurate understanding of why they need to make a change to their health behaviours
- Encourage individuals to begin to think about changing behaviour, not convince them that they have to change (Zimmerman 2000)
- People not yet contemplating change will not respond to traditional interventions or behavioural programmes. They require specific input to increase their awareness of the importance of recommendations. MI can be used to explore attitudes around behaviour change (Hammond et al. 2004)
- This earlier motivational phase is about raising awareness and empowering individuals to take control. It is when the level of motivation or intention reaches a particular level that the individual is assumed to be likely to move on to later stages (Diclemente et al. 1991)
- Advising individuals about what action to take towards behaviour change is misdirected in this stage and can often result in the individuals becoming defensive resulting in resistance (Rollnick et al. 1992)

Adapted from Ogden (2011).

Therapeutic interventions to promote health behaviour change

- Edward may be resistant to changing his routine; therefore, it is important to work with this resistance and explore his ambivalence rather than trying to push him into action (Keefe et al. 2000).
- Emphasise that it is up to him whether or not he changes his work routine.
- Consciousness raising – provide *small* amounts of information about the elements of his work routine that can exacerbate his RA to increase his understanding.
- Explore ideas around making a change to his working routine using MI (Table 7.2).

Table 7.2   The contemplation stage of the TTM.

Stage of change	Characteristics
Contemplation Intention to make a change to their behaviours in the foreseeable future, but feel ambivalent about what this change will involve	Individuals maybe beginning to be aware that they may need to change their health behaviours, but still feel undecided and question what they have to gain from making any changes, therefore they remain ambivalent
Processes of change to encourage health behaviour change	
• *Self re-evaluation* – encourage individuals to assess the pros and cons of making a health behaviour change • Highlight the barriers to change and look at ways to overcome these to increase the individuals motivation • Focus on exploring and increasing readiness to change and self-efficacy	

Adapted from Ogden (2011).

Contemplation

> Today I feel not too bad and yet if I do any work it's so frustrating I sit here and I feel all right but as soon as I do anything the next day I suffer.

- Edward was used to being very active and was feeling frustrated about the things he now found difficult.
- He was exploring what he had to gain; he felt it was a choice between doing too much manual labour and paying for it afterwards, or giving into the condition and losing control. This is a familiar feeling for individuals with rheumatic conditions (Magem 2010).
- He was trying to cover up his difficulties from his brothers because he did not want to worry them. McArthur (2002) highlighted that individuals often chose not to inform individuals at their workplace of their biomechanical disruptions until they have no choice.

Therapeutic interventions to promote health behaviour change

- Self-re-evaluation – Encourage Edward to consider the pros or cons of discussing his work struggles with his brothers. The aim is to encourage him to recognise the potential benefits of his brothers carrying out the heavier tasks on the farm, and also to identify any barriers.
- Self-monitoring – Ask him to keep records of his key symptoms (pain, fatigue, joint swelling) and their severity when carrying out certain physical tasks on the farm. Encourage him to recognise how those tasks can exacerbate his symptoms to increase his motivation to change (Keefe et al. 2000).
- Explore how convinced he is that changing his work routine could decrease his symptoms. The focus is to help him to understand that a change in routine

Table 7.3 The preparation stage of the TTM.

Stage of change	Characteristics
Preparation	
Acknowledgement that there are more pros to making a behaviour change than cons	Individuals have made a commitment to change and are now making plans on how to implement the changes
Processes of change to encourage health behaviour change	
• *Commitment* – Identify the skills and knowledge that the individual has and what they require to resume responsibility of the change • Adopt a graded approach to identify small steps towards change to increase commitment. It is important to assist individuals in making a conscious commitment to change and adapt their behaviours • Develop problem-solving techniques to overcome barriers and obstacles for the individuals	

Adapted from Ogden (2011).

could have a positive effect, thereby enhancing his internal LOC and sense of self-efficacy.

- Reassure him that he is not losing control and empower him to take control in managing his rheumatic condition.
- It is unlikely he will accept any equipment to assist with joint protection; therefore, a problem-solving approach is indicated (Table 7.3).

Preparation

My lower back pain does improve slightly when my workload is reduced...

- Edward acknowledged that there were more pros than cons to making a change to his work routine and informing his brothers of his struggles.

Therapeutic interventions to promote health behaviour change

- Commitment – Use Specific, Measurable, Achievable, Realistic and Timely (SMART) goals with Edward to plan how he will implement the changes to his work routine and how he will inform his brother about these changes. SMART goals are more likely to be client-centred and achievable (Randall and McEwan 2000).
- Set dates to implement these changes to enhance commitment.
- Encourage him to seek support from family and friends to promote change.
- Identify small changes that can minimise fatigue and pain to enable him to feel the benefits of his behaviour changes, for example (a) looking at his sleep hygiene and (b) suggesting that his brothers complete the early morning tasks as Edward had significant early morning stiffness (EMS). Encourage him to reflect on the potential benefits of these changes.

Table 7.4   The action stage of the TTM.

Stage of change	Characteristics
Action Changes starting to happen	Individuals have made some overt changes to modify their behaviour and are continuing to make notable overt efforts to change They are taking control and feel a greater internal LoC
Processes of change to encourage health behaviour change	
• *Countering* – Confidence-building techniques to encourage the individual to focus on the positives of the changes they have made. Looking at healthy coping strategies here to relieve stress and anxiety that maybe experienced in the initial stages of implementing the change • Social support important to reinforce behaviour change • Individuals need strategies to maintain the behaviour • Focus on supporting and increasing self-efficacy further • People in the action stage can experience lower levels of weekly pain (Strand et al. 2007)	

Adapted from Ogden (2011).

- Plan coping strategies with Edward. Initially, he may experience high levels of stress and anxiety with this change to his daily routine. Explore the use of mindfulness (see Chapter 6) to minimise this as bringing the mind back to the present moment increases clarity, calmness and well-being. Mindfulness aims to help individuals to notice and relate differently to thoughts and feelings, and this could be particularly useful for Edward to manage his anxieties around change.
- Discuss self-management tips that Edward can adopt to help him feel in control (Table 7.4).

Action

  I've got two brothers that now do some of the heavier work.

- Edward has made changes to his workload; his brothers now milk the cows and complete the routine heavy tasks on the farm whilst Edward takes on work that avoids early morning starts (because of his EMS) and late afternoons (when he is particularly tired).

Therapeutic interventions to promote health behaviour change

- Review Edward's work routine and complete task analysis to identify any further activities to change.
- Encourage him to evaluate the internal rewards experienced since changing his work routine and to discuss this with his support network.
- He may be feeling better physically; therefore, it is important to reinforce the importance of continuing with the changes he has made and not reverting back to his old work routine.
- Continue to encourage self-efficacy (Table 7.5).

Table 7.5   The maintenance stage of the TTM.

Stage of change	Characteristics
Maintenance Maintaining change	Individuals have sustained overt changes over time for a minimum of 6 months and are consolidating and integrating these changes into their daily lifeOccasional lapses may occur but overall behaviour is sustained
Processes of change to encourage health behaviour change	
• *Relapse prevention* – encourage individuals to seek the rewards of self-management to continue motivation and self-efficacy	

Adapted from Ogden (2011).

Maintenance

My brothers have been completing the routine heavy duty tasks in the mornings and late afternoons now for the past six months....

• Edward has been maintaining the health behaviour changes for over 6 months.

Therapeutic interventions to promote health behaviour change

• Follow-up with Edward and encourage him to continue to self-monitor his symptoms as he may need to make further changes to his work routine as his condition progresses.

7.9   Limitations of the TTM

• *Does not consider social aspects of certain behaviours and the impact this can have on change*. Therefore, it is useful to consider the social influences highlighted by the TPB and ensure a holistic approach is used to identify any social influences that can impact on an individual's readiness to change.
• *People can move through the stages quickly making it difficult to assess an individual's stage*. Assessing the stage of change that an individual is in is an ongoing process. Having an awareness of the key characteristics of the different stages can inform occupational therapists' assessments and so inform clinical reasoning.
• *Individuals can be in different stages for different aspects of managing their rheumatic condition*. Individuals cannot be put into one stage of change for all aspects of their self-management. It is important to explore the different aspects of self-management and explore the stage of change the individual is in for these different aspects. Occupational therapist can then target these aspects individually.

7.10   Conclusion

Individuals with rheumatic conditions are encouraged to make lifestyle changes to assist with the self-management of their long-term condition. Occupational therapists can incorporate their understanding of behavioural change theory to enhance client-centred practice by tailoring interventions to match the stage of change that individuals are in. This promotes behaviour change and encourages individuals to more effectively self-manage their rheumatic conditions.

Resources

Department of Health Guidelines for Promoting Behaviour Change. http://www.dh.gov.uk/en/Publicationsandstatistics/Publications/PublicationsPolicyAndGuidance/DH_085779. Accessed on 14 November 2012.

Information on Factors to Consider When Helping Individuals with Long-Term Conditions to Make Changes to Health Behaviours. https://tools.skillsforhealth.org.uk/competence/show/html/id/1847/. Accessed on 14 November 2012.

NICE Guideline for Behavioural Change. http://www.nice.org.uk/PH6. Accessed on 14 November 2012.

University of Rhode Island Change Assessment: A 32-item self-report questionnaire to assess stages of adoption of self-management. It can be used to measure how much individuals are considering making behavioural changes to cope with their arthritis. http://www.painjournalonline.com/article/S0304-3959(00)00294-3/abstract. Accessed on 14 November 2012.

References

Burg J, Conner C, Harre N, et al. (2005) The trans-theoretical model and stages of change: A critique observations by five commentators on the paper by Adams J and Whire M (2004) Why don't stage based activity promotion interventions work? *Health Education Research* 20(2):244–258.

Davis P, Busch A, Lowe JC, et al. (1994) Evaluation of a rheumatoid arthritis patient education programme impact on knowledge and self efficacy. *Patient Education and Counselling* 24:55–61.

DiClemente CC, Hughes SO (1990) Stages of change profiles in outpatient alcoholism treatment. *Journal of Substance Abuse* 2(2):217–235.

DiClemente CC, Prochaska JO, Fairhurst SK, et al. (1991) The process of smoking cessation: An analysis of pre-contemplation, contemplation, and preparation stages of change. *Journal of Consulting and Clinical Psychology* 59(2):295–304.

Dubouloz CJ, Vallerand J, Laporte D, et al. (2008) Occupational performance modification and personal change among clients receiving rehabilitation services for rheumatoid arthritis. *Australian Occupational Therapy Journal* 55:30–38.

Freeman KE, Hammond A, Lincoln NB (2002) Use of cognitive-behavioural arthritis education programmes in newly diagnosed rheumatoid arthritis. *Clinical Rehabilitation* 16:828–836.

Goodacre LG, Goodacre JA (2004) Factors influencing the beliefs of patients with rheumatoid arthritis regarding disease modifying medication. *Rheumatology* 43(5):583–586.

Hammond A, Lincoln N, Sutcliffe L (1999) A crossover trail evaluating an educational-behavioural joint protection programme for people with rheumatoid arthritis. *Patient Education and Counseling* 37:19–32.

Hammond A, Young A, Kidao R (2004) A randomised controlled trial of occupational therapy for people with early rheumatoid arthritis. *Annals of Rheumatic Diseases* 63(1):23–30.

Keefe FJ, Lefebvre JC, Kerns R, et al. (2000) Understanding the adoption of self management: Stages of change profiles among arthritis patients. *Pain* 8(3):303–313.

Kerns RD, Rosenberg R (2000) Predicting responses to self management treatments for chronic pain: Application of the stages of change model. *Pain* 84(1):49–55.

Magem S (2010) Reflections on inflammatory arthritis. *The Journal of Rheumatology Occupational Therapy* 25(1):11–13.

Maio GR, Haddock G (2009) *The Psychology of Attitudes and Attitude Change*. London: Sage Publications Ltd.

McArthur MA (2002) *Unheard Stories, Unmet Needs: The Clinical and Educational Implications of Perceptions of Rheumatoid Arthritis*. Ph.D. thesis, Centre for Applied Research in Education, School of Education and Professional Development, University of East Anglia, Norfolk, UK.

McPherson KM, Brander P, Taylor WJ, et al. (2001) Living with arthritis: What is important? *Disability and Rehabilitation* 23(16):706–721.

Miller K (2005) *Communications Theories: Perspectives, Processes, and Contexts*. New York: McGraw-Hill.

Miller WR, Rollnick S (2002) *Motivational Interviewing: Preparing People for Change* (2nd edn.). New York: Guildford Press.

Morrison V, Bennett P (2009) *An Introduction to Health Psychology* (2nd edn.). Harlow, UK: Pearson Education Ltd.

Ogden J (2011) *Health Psychology: A Textbook* (4th edn.). England, UK: Open University Press.

Pradhan E, Baumgarten M, Langenberg P, et al. (2007) Effect of mindfulness-based stress reduction in rheumatoid arthritis patients. *Arthritis Care and Research* 57(7):1134–1142.

Randall KE, McEwan IR (2000) Writing patient centred functional goals. *Physical Therapy* 80(12):1197–1203.

Rollnick S, Heather N, Bell A (1992) Negotiating behaviour change in medical settings: The development of brief motivational interviewing. *Journal of Mental Health* 1(1):25–37.

Strand EB, Kerns RD, Christle A, et al. (2007) Higher levels of pain readiness to change and more positive affect reduce pain reports – A weekly assessment study on arthritis. *Pain* 127(3):204–213.

Taol E, Rasker JJ, Wiegman O (1996) Patient education and self management in the rheumatic diseases: A self efficacy approach. *American College of Rheumatology* 9(3):229–238.

Thirlaway K, Upton D (2009) *The Psychology of Lifestyle: Promoting Healthy Behaviour*. London: Routledge, Taylor & Francis Group.

Weinstein N (1984) Why it won't happen to me: Perceptions of risk factors and susceptibility. *Health Psychology* 3:431–457.

Zimmerman GL, Olsen CG, Bosworth MF (2007) A stages of change approach to helping patients change behaviour. *American Family Physician* 61(5):1409–1416.

Chapter 8

Joint protection

Alison Hammond

Centre for Health Sciences Research, University of Salford, Salford, United Kingdom

8.1 Introduction

Many people with arthritis and musculoskeletal conditions (MSCs) can find many of their everyday activities painful, tiring and frustrating, affecting their well-being.

Joint protection is not just a physical intervention. It is an active coping strategy to improve daily tasks and role performance, reduce frustration, enhance perceptions of control and improve psychological status (Hammond et al. 1999).

This chapter discusses what joint protection is; aims and principles; why and when to use it; what people with arthritis understand and perceive joint protection to be; what facilitates or prevents them applying joint protection in daily life; evidence for joint protection effectiveness; how to provide effective joint protection education to facilitate behaviour change; and some joint protection techniques. Because hand function is often disrupted in arthritis and MSCs, much joint protection literature focuses on the hands. Joint protection in rheumatoid arthritis (RA) will be a particular focus in this chapter.

8.2 What is joint protection?

Joint protection is a core component of rheumatology occupational therapy underlying the rehabilitation of all people whose joints are at risk from arthritis (Cordery and Rocchi 1998). It includes:

- altering working methods,
- use of proper joint and body mechanics,

Rheumatology Practice in Occupational Therapy: Promoting Lifestyle Management, First Edition.
Edited by Lynne Goodacre and Margaret McArthur.

- using assistive devices,
- modifying activities and routines,
- pacing activities and
- modifying environments.

Therefore, it is the application of ergonomics in daily activities, work and leisure (Hammond 2010). It is often integrated with fatigue management, hand exercises and provision of working splints (see also Chapters 9 and 12). It was first developed in the 1960s (Cordery 1965) applying understanding of the pathophysiology of joint diseases, biomechanics, forces applied during activity and how deformities develop (Brattstrom 1987; Chamberlain et al. 1984; Cordery 1965; Cordery and Rocchi 1998; Melvin 1989). Whilst first developed for people with RA, its use has extended into many other MSCs in which people experience joint or soft tissue pain and swelling (Brattstrom 1987; Chamberlain et al. 1984; Cordery and Rocchi 1998; Melvin 1989; Sheon 1985).

8.3   The aims of joint protection

In inflammatory arthritis the aims of joint protection are to:

- reduce pain during activity and at rest resulting from pressure on nociceptive endings in joint capsules from inflammation and mechanical forces on joints,
- reduce forces on joints: internal (i.e. from muscular compressive forces, e.g. during strong grip) or external (i.e. forces applied to joints whilst carrying or pulling/ pushing objects),
- help preserve joint integrity and reduce risk of development and/or progression of deformities,
- reduce fatigue by reducing effort required for activity performance and
- improve or maintain function.

For people with osteoarthritis (OA), the aims are to:

- reduce loading on articular cartilage and subchondral bone,
- strengthen muscle support and
- improve shock-absorbing capabilities of joints (Cordery and Rocchi 1998).

For people with soft tissue disorders, the aims are to reduce:

- pain,
- inflammation and
- strain on soft tissues (Sheon 1985).

8.4   Why and when to use joint protection

Joint protection is designed as a preventative strategy. In inflammatory arthropathies (and some other MSCs), inflammation increases intra-articular pressure, which, in the short term, results in pain. Longer-term, persistent synovitis gradually causes capsular and ligamentous laxity and erosions of subchondral bone. Combined with both normal and abnormal forces passing over joints, these factors increase the risk of deformities developing (Adams et al. 2005; Flatt 1995). Synovitis arises from the disease process. However, most people with arthritis recognise that when they 'overuse' their joints, forcing themselves to keep going through pain and fatigue, synovitis increases, lasts longer and they are in pain and fatigued for longer. These symptoms contribute to less efficient ways of working and poorer body mechanics, compounding problems.

Joint protection works in tandem with medication, which reduces synovitis and pain, to reduce the additional component of joint swelling arising from 'overuse'. Remember, 'overuse' for someone with arthritis generally equates to a normal level of use for a person without arthritis. It can be psychologically difficult for those with arthritis to accept the fluctuating boundaries of what they can comfortably do on any one day, meaning that 'overuse' for them can change daily.

Exercise also contributes to 'protecting' joints. Stronger muscles do not tire as easily, slowing onset of muscle aching, and help to support joints with capsular and ligamentous laxity. Fatigue management (e.g. energy conservation, relaxation, sleep hygiene, stress management) increases available energy to expend in exercise and physical activity, enhancing muscle strength and endurance and thus helping protect joints (Figure 8.1).

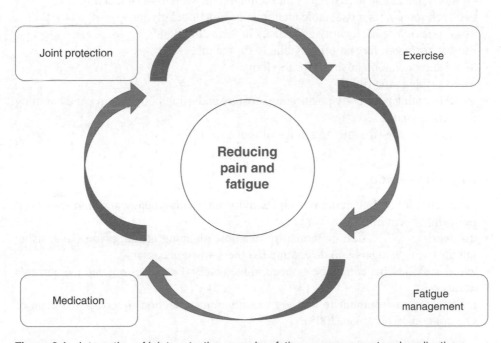

Figure 8.1 Interaction of joint protection, exercise, fatigue management and medication.

In consequence, joint protection should be applied from an early stage to reduce inflammation and forces on joints disrupted by the disease process. If applied later, it will still help reduce pain but, if joint disruption has already occurred, longer term it reduces the opportunity to limit this. Given that joint protection involves altering habitual movement patterns and methods of activity performance, changing habits and routines permanently is more effective than a stop-start approach. It is easy to forget to use joint protection. Indeed, in the early stages of learning joint protection methods, many say they remembered to use them after the action or activity, when they were already in pain.

8.5　Joint protection and energy conservation principles

Different authors have identified a variety of principles. A consensus was published by the College of Occupational Therapy Specialist Section in Rheumatology (COT 2003):

Joint protection

- respect pain: use this as a signal to change activities,
- distribute load over several joints,
- reduce the force and effort required to perform activities by altering working methods, using assistive devices and reducing the weight of objects,
- use each joint in its most stable anatomic or functional plane,
- avoid positions of deformity and forces in their direction,
- use the strongest, largest joint available for the job,
- avoid staying in one position for too long,
- avoid gripping too tightly,
- avoid adopting poor body positioning, posture and using poor moving and handling techniques and
- maintain muscle strength and range of movement.

Energy conservation

- pace activities by balancing rest and activity, alternating heavy and light tasks and performing activities more slowly,
- use work simplification methods, for example planning ahead, prioritising, using labour saving gadgets and delegating to others when necessary,
- avoid activities that cannot be stopped immediately if it proves beyond the person's ability and
- modify the environment to suit ergonomic/joint protection practices (College of Occupational Therapists 2003).

See Chapter 10 for further information on energy conservation.

8.6   Understanding and perceptions of joint protection

In a study of people with RA for on average 13 (SD 9.97) years (*n* = 10), most understood correctly what joint protection is:

a specific way of performing a task to help make activities easier, holding joint(s) physically in the right position, maintaining joint function through exercise; keeping pain to a minimum; not working until fatigued or overusing, as fatigue leads to false positioning.

But some had inappropriate ideas:

do not use the joints, use as few as possible; only during certain activities or when its especially important; only when pain is present.

One considered it 'like an obligation, like you have to' and another with earlier stage disease that 'I often avoid [doing] joint protection and think it's not yet necessary'. Others with more established disease explained how their use of joint protection increased with their acceptance of and coping with arthritis.

'At the beginning of the disease it was less important. The longer the duration, the more important it is. One realizes it is necessary and helpful' and 'if something is useful, it doesn't matter what other people think' (Niedermann et al. 2010a, b, p. 150).

The term 'joint protection' can thus be misunderstood, considered as 'giving in', stopping activities, keeping joints immobile and resting excessively. As one person with RA described it, 'it's wrapping yourself up in cotton wool, isn't it?' (Hammond and Lincoln 1999a). An important first step in joint protection education is therefore being clear about what it is and is not. Many with arthritis and MSCs (and some health professionals) find it confusing that the occupational therapist teaches people to 'protect joints' (incorrectly interpreted as limiting movement and activity) whilst the physiotherapist tells them to exercise as much as possible (incorrectly interpreted as doing exercise which will cause pain and strain). In the earlier stages of a condition, when the person is adjusting to living with it, this apparent contradiction is puzzling and may lead to people doing neither.

Benefits of joint protection

People with RA consistently emphasised the physical and psychological benefits of joint protection (Niedermann et al. 2010a, b). These were improved:

- Physical well-being: resulting from less pain and better function. 'I can avoid pain…and reduce pain that is present; it is easier for me to perform routine physical tasks; I have less physical stress; I have more strength'.
- Psychological well-being: 'I have more energy for friends and family; I feel less stressed; it puts me in a better mood for the rest of the day; it helps me have a more positive outlook on life'.
- Potential benefits were seen as 'I can prevent damage; I have a higher quality of life; I am more relaxed in the longer term; and I save later health costs for the healthcare system'.

- Personal control: 'it makes me feel more confident; I can actively contribute to my health; I feel more independent from other people; I can take better care of my joints'.
- Self-acceptance: 'I feel good about myself if I keep my commitment to look after my joints regularly; I am more content with myself'.

Barriers to joint protection

Participants in this study also identified barriers, but reported that these mainly occurred in the earlier stages of the disease. They subsequently considered them as potential barriers for others, but no longer for themselves. Having accepted using joint protection they had overcome the two key barriers of:

- The negative impact on self-image: 'feeling uncomfortable or embarrassed using assistive devices; feeling dependent on the use of assistive devices; doing things differently gives me the image of feeling disabled; I am afraid to attract attention'.
- The difficulty and effort involved: 'there is too much effort to learn to do it correctly; the tasks are more time consuming; it is unusual and that can lead to tension; I have to make more of an effort'.

Thus, especially in the earlier stages people with arthritis or MSCs may be reluctant to change how they do everyday activities and concerned that they may 'have to give up things they like doing'. This can affect their sense of self, as our occupations contribute to our sense of identity. The early, negative effect of using assistive devices on self-image was particularly highlighted. People want to feel normal, not set themselves apart from others by acting differently. They may prefer to persevere through pain because psychologically, accepting the change to one's sense of self may be worse than the pain.

8.7   Goals of joint protection education

These include facilitating people to make:

(a) Cognitive change: understanding the why, what, how, when and where of using joint protection.
(b) Attitudinal and affective change: this includes enabling the person to develop a degree of acceptance or emotional adjustment to the condition; increasing their internal locus of control, i.e. believing that the use of joint protection can make a difference; increasing their belief in the benefits of using joint protection; increasing their self-efficacy; increasing their willingness to change habits and routines to use joint protection; and their motivation or intention to adhere with using it in future.
(c) Behavioural change: adopting and maintaining joint protection at an appropriate frequency to make a difference to health. This requires the appropriate level of psychomotor skill.

All three goals need to be addressed for education to lead successfully to health status changes. Joint protection cannot be effective if insufficient behavioural change occurs. Providing verbal and written information and demonstrating joint protection methods may help people make cognitive but not necessarily attitudinal and behavioural changes. Therefore different strategies are required.

8.8   Evidence for joint protection effectiveness

Many attempts to change behaviour by making a change in knowledge (traditional handouts, demonstration, discussions) have been largely unsuccessful. Using cognitive, behavioural and learning theories to develop teaching programmes have been effective (Cordery and Rocchi 1998, p. 316).

Usual joint protection education

Commonly, occupational therapists teach joint protection over one to two sessions, for on average 1.5 h. This includes explaining how joints are affected by the condition, the rationale for and principles of joint protection, demonstrations of some techniques and short supervised practice (for at most 30 min). Several randomised controlled trials (RCTs) have evaluated this format, either provided one-to-one or as part of group arthritis education programmes. Knowledge improved in these but not use of joint protection (Barry et al. 1994; Hammond and Freeman 2001; Hammond and Lincoln 1999a). In the latter study, three months after education, over half of the participants (with RA for 6.43 (SD 7.7) years; $n = 21$) interviewed considered they had made few or no changes. Barriers to change were:

- difficulty recalling methods (insufficient cognitive change),
- joint protection was not considered necessary as 'my hands are not that bad yet' or they used techniques 'on bad days only' (insufficient attitudinal change) and
- difficulty getting used to the different actions, which felt 'clumsy and slow', they seemed more effort than normal and difficulty 'changing the habits of a lifetime' (insufficient psychomotor skills and behavioural change).

The remaining participants considered they had made changes. However, video analysis of hand-use patterns before and after education showed that many changes described were already being used before education. Education had raised awareness of changes already made but was probably of insufficient duration to address attitudinal and behavioural changes.

Behavioural joint protection education in RA

In contrast, structured group programmes, of 8–16 h duration, emphasising active learning, problem solving, behavioural approaches, frequent practice and home programmes have been proven to be effective. An RCT with people with early RA ($n = 127$) compared an 8-h joint protection programme (the 'Looking After Your Joints Programme (LAJP)'), with a standard arthritis education programme, including 2.5 h of usual joint protection (i.e. similar to that described earlier). The LAJP applied cognitive behavioural, educational and motor learning approaches to promote change. At 1 year, the LAJP group had significantly increased use of joint protection, better functional ability and less hand pain, general pain and early morning stiffness (Hammond and Freeman 2001). At 4 years, the LAJP group continued to have significantly greater adherence with joint protection, better function and less early morning stiffness than the standard education group. The LAJP group also had significantly fewer hand deformities (Hammond and Freeman 2004). The original LAJP focused only on joint protection, as the aim of the trial was to evaluate whether joint protection was effective. Having demonstrated this, the LAJP has now been extended to include fatigue management and hand exercises, plus splint provision if this is identified as appropriate. The revised LAJP can now be delivered as a stand-alone module or as one of two modules in the Lifestyle Management for Arthritis Programme (LMAP) (Hammond et al. 2008).

An RCT, of four sessions of joint protection provided one-to-one, with a similar theory base, teaching methods and content as the LAJP, at three months follow-up, also led to significantly improved use of joint protection and self-efficacy (Niedermann et al. 2011). A key element was the individualisation of the programme content, achieved by using the Pictorial Representation of Illness and Self-Measure (PRISM) and PRISM+ assessment method (Buchi et al. 1998). This is a hands-on tool in which the person moves coloured discs (representative of their illness, life and important aspects of the person's life) closer or further away from the disc representing self. This helps in identifying meaningful occupations, promoting discussion of these, how joint protection can help and motivation to use it.

Joint protection combined with other interventions in RA

Several RCTs have been conducted of combined interventions. At eight month follow-up, a 12-h programme of joint protection, exercise, cognitive pain management and relaxation, with monthly telephone follow-up, led to significant improvements in pain, functional ability and physical status. Participants ($n = 70$) had established RA (average 15 years) and were all on stable biologic therapy. The intervention thus provided gains over and above the effects of biologic therapy (Masiero et al. 2007).

The LMAP comprises module 1 of the LAJP, a second module 'Keeping Mobile' (exercise, pain and stress management) and a booster session. At 1 year follow-up, in people with established RA on stable drug therapy ($n = 167$), the LMAP group significantly improved pain, functional and physical ability, self-efficacy and psychological status compared to a group receiving standard arthritis education (Hammond et al. 2008).

Joint protection in hand OA

Several RCTs of joint protection in hand OA have been conducted. At three month follow-up, a combined programme of joint protection and hand exercises led to significant improvements in grip strength and self-perceived hand function (Stamm et al. 2002). At 6-month follow-up, a hand joint protection intervention (based on the LAJP) led to significant improvements in the numbers of participants meeting responder criteria (i.e. a combination of hand pain, hand disability and global improvement) and self-efficacy (Dziedzic et al. 2011a,b). At 1 year follow-up, a combined programme of joint protection, hand exercises and splinting led to significant improvements in pain, stiffness and daily activities (Boustedt et al. 2009).

8.9 The Looking After Your Joints Programme and the Lifestyle Management for Arthritis Programme

A recent systematic review identified that common features of effective self-management interventions are those that explicitly use social cognitive theory and/or cognitive-behavioural therapy approaches; enable participants to develop individualised weekly action plans with progress review; and are highly protocolised with leader manuals and participant workbooks (Iversen et al. 2010).

These approaches have been integrated into the LAJP (Hammond and Freeman 2001, 2004) and the LMAP (Hammond 2012; Hammond et al. 2008). Both have leader manuals and participant workbooks, have been tested in RCTs and proven effective. The modular approach allows people to make changes gradually. Providing joint protection to six clients in the 10-h LAJP is at little extra cost to treating six clients for 1.5 h individually. The LAJP is more effective as each client receives significantly more therapy plus the highly valued opportunity to learn and gain support from each other.

8.10 Teaching joint protection

This section discusses how the theoretical and practical approaches are combined within the LAJP and LMAP. These approaches can equally be applied in individual joint protection education. Further information about the theory and techniques included in these two programmes has also been published elsewhere (Hammond 2003, 2010; Hammond and Niedermann 2010).

Applying the Transtheoretical Model to joint protection

Effective joint protection education requires firstly identifying the person's readiness to change. Identifying their pros and cons or benefits and barriers, both practical and psychological, of using joint protection will assist in determining how best to facilitate the person to change. As described in Chapter 7, the Transtheoretical Model (TTM) identifies that people cycle through a series of *five stages of change* when modifying health behaviours (Prochaska and DiClemente 1992).

During the initial assessment with the client, the therapist will have identified which joints and/or soft tissues are affected, symptom severity (e.g. pain, fatigue), the effect of the condition on daily activities, work and leisure and the client's priorities for treatment. During this interview, the therapist can ask, for example:

- 'What do you currently do to help manage how your pain?' and 'Does fatigue affect your ability to do the activities you need and want to do in life?'

Their response will help identify what stage of change they may be in. The TTM recommends different approaches and interventions for each stage to help people progress. In the lower stages (1–3), cognitive and affective strategies are important, whereas in the upper stages (4 and 5) behavioural processes are most important.

Stages 1 and 2: pre-contemplation and contemplation

If the person is not yet ready to make changes, changing attitudes by providing small amounts of information incrementally is the priority before teaching practical skills. Explore what activities and roles are important to the person, if they are affected by arthritis, what difficulties result (e.g. pain, fatigue, stiffness, frustration) and concerns for the future. A technique used in motivational interviewing is to ask:

- How important is it for you to reduce these symptoms and continue these activities, on a scale of 0–10?
- How confident do you feel about making changes on a scale of 0–10?
- How ready are you to make changes on a scale of 0–10?

0 is not at all important, confident or ready and 10 extremely important, confident and ready (Mason and Butler 2010).

If their score is less than 7 for any of these, they are less likely to see the need for or be willing to change. If this is the case: explore what they think might increase these beliefs and their confidence in and readiness to use joint protection; explain that joint protection and fatigue management are proven to be effective and discuss the benefits that can be gained (i.e. reduced pain and fatigue, staying independent, less frustration, better physical and psychological well-being); allow time for the person to discuss their concerns about negative self-image, embarrassment, not wanting to use assistive devices, wanting to remain as they are, not wanting to take the time to change, concerns that joint protection is slower and more difficult (Niedermann et al. 2010a).

Consider how to 'market' joint protection. 'Looking after your joints' and 'applying ergonomics' means adapting activities and movements to reduce strain or force on joints and soft tissues. Using altered working methods, planning, pacing and restructuring activities are less obvious changes to people than using devices and splints. Emphasise how many techniques are similar to those widely used in industry to reduce physical strain and injury risk and enable people to work more efficiently. Less pain and fatigue means one has the energy and physical ability to do more things one enjoys or wants to keep on doing in life, such as working, playing with the children and going out socially. Care should be taken that joint protection is not perceived as 'not' doing things and appearing different. The use of assistive devices should be introduced gradually as the person is more accepting of change. Joint protection should be promoted as, longer term, helping people to continue with or get back to doing valued activities and participating in meaningful roles.

Change is a choice. The person may have good reasons for not using joint protection and energy conservation strategies at a specific time. There may be other priorities to be managed first: new medication; work; childcare; increasing exercise; counselling. clients' priorities include remaining in control of their condition, which paradoxically can include not wanting interventions even when recognising their importance (Ward et al. 2007). Tell people they can come back at any time if they would like more information and provide written information (e.g. Arthritis Research UK's *Looking After Your Joints* booklet 2011). Ensure there are regular opportunities for people to be re-referred. Recognise when it is appropriate not to provide joint protection education, which also assists service efficiency.

Stage 3: preparation

In this stage, the pros for joint protection are more compelling and the advantages of change are considered with taking action being planned for the near future (i.e. within a month). Small steps are being taken that they believe can help them make joint protection part of their lives (e.g. telling others they want to change). It is important to identify the joint protection knowledge and skills they already have and those they need to develop and to provide appropriate information about what and how to do joint protection.

Self-monitoring can be encouraged through observing one's behaviours, evaluating if pain or fatigue is less when practising a joint protection method and evaluating if the change is beneficial.

Avoid promoting overambitious goals too soon and teach problem-solving skills. Engaging family and friends in planning joint protection changes, buying assistive devices as presents and reading joint protection advice leaflets can also be helpful.

Stages 4 and 5: action and maintenance

In stage 4, activities are being performed to modify joint protection behaviours and adapt the environment, leading to an increasing sense of competence and control in using joint protection. A person may look to others for support to continue to change. This stage lasts about 6 months and can include lapses and lead to relapse. A coaching and educational-behavioural approach can be used in stage 4 to teach joint protection principles and their application across different activities; motor learning approaches with sufficient supervised practice and feedback can help psychomotor skill development; task analysis can enable a person to identify actions and activities to change; problem-solving can enable a person to apply joint protection principles to generate new solutions and help overcome barriers and prevent lapses; goal-setting can enable a person to regularly set and review action plans and how to identify internal rewards for meeting these. Workbooks, diaries and action plans can help recall of information and recording activities, joint protection behaviours practiced and intentions to change.

It is important to increase and support self-efficacy by collaboratively developing home programmes to promote joint protection. This can also be achieved through facilitating social support at home and work and encourage buddying up of clients for mutual support.

In stage 5, new joint protection behaviours are consolidated and integrated into daily life with occasional lapses still occurring. Follow-up support should be planned, for example booster sessions, and progress should be reviewed annually. People need to be made aware of the risk of reverting to old habits and how to cope with lapses.

The TTM identifies that stages 1 and 2 are associated with lower levels of self-efficacy (i.e. confidence in ability to perform the action) and stages 4 and 5 progressively associated with higher levels of self-efficacy (see also Chapter 7).

Social cognitive theory applied to joint protection

Enhancing self-efficacy for joint protection is a key element of teaching joint protection. Strategies to enhance self-efficacy include (Bandura 1977):

(a) Mastery experience: i.e. performing tasks successfully. Changing automatic movement habits and embedded daily routines has been identified by clients as one of the major barriers to change. It is essential to provide sufficient practice of skills, with feedback, starting with simpler and moving to more complex skills.
(b) Vicarious experience (role modelling): watching others like ourselves successfully perform actions enhances our beliefs that we can also succeed. Teaching joint protection in groups enables modelling, joint problem-solving, peer support and exchange of ideas.
(c) Verbal persuasion: i.e. encouraging the person to try skills. Although widely used by health professionals, providing direct and vicarious experiences are more effective. Persuasion should be an adjunct to these.
(d) Reinterpretation of physiological signals: helping people perceive the difference between disease symptoms and, for example, increased symptoms (aches, fatigue, joint swelling) due to overdoing activities. Therefore, symptoms can be partly controlled through joint protection and fatigue management.

Cognitive-behavioural approaches and goal-setting in joint protection

Change is the person's responsibility. The therapist's responsibility is providing effective interventions which enable the person to change. Goal-setting and action plans aid effective self-management. Identifying long-term goals aids motivation, for example maintaining meaningful activities and how using joint protection helps achieve these (e.g. being able to stay at work). Whilst supervised practice with a therapist aids correct skill development, continued practice at home is essential for habit development.

Short-term goals, towards achieving long-term goals, should state: what, how much, when, how often and the time frame. An example of an action plan is included in Figure 8.2. Plans must be achievable. A simple way of checking this is to ask how confident the person is about achieving, on a scale of 0–10, (a) each goal and (b) the whole plan. If their answer falls below 7 for any or all, then the plan should be revised to be achievable. Lorig et al. (2007) include a user-friendly approach to goal-setting.

Each education session should include setting goals until the next session. At the beginning of each session, progress in meeting these goals should be discussed, with appropriate positive feedback or supportive discussion and problem-solving to reduce barriers if any were not met.

Educational approaches in joint protection

Effective teaching requires forward planning to enable joint protection knowledge and skills development. The environment should be comfortable and free of distracting noise. Audio-visual aids are best kept simple. Many people are not familiar with teaching and training environments. Using PowerPoint can make sessions seem more formal and people often watch the screen rather than the therapist or other group members. A pre-prepared flip-chart or A3 Easel presenter/portfolio, placed on the table, with pre-printed sheets is cheap, less formal, quicker to set up and very unlikely to go wrong. Group comments can be added to spare sheets, and it is easily updated as teaching topics change.

Recall of information can be improved by use of:

- Simplification: have a few key messages each session. Explain technical terms when necessary (e.g. inflammation) and use non-technical words (e.g. bend not flex). Keep explanations short.
- Explicit categorisation: structure information to 'tell them what you are going to tell them, tell them, and tell them what you told them'. Summarise pre- and post- each topic, and at the beginning and end of the session overall. This helps people retain information more readily.
- Repetition: ensure key facts are repeated by paraphrasing, and asking the person to repeat back or paraphrase what they have learnt. Repetition is an important component of education: both of facts and skills.

Psychomotor skills teaching applied to joint protection

Developing psychomotor skills requires the formation of new mental schemas or movement patterns (Schmidt and Lee 2005). When teaching skills, four stages can be followed (Mackway-Jones and Walker (1999):

1 Layout: Plan for sufficient space; ensure there are no obstacles. Check client/s can see clearly. Furniture, equipment or people may need to be moved.
2 Equipment: Ensure all required is to hand, the therapist is totally familiar with its use. Anything not immediately required should be put aside to avoid visual distraction.

Dates from:___Monday_____ to:_____Sunday_____	

The Plan:

1. Practise the flexibility and strength hand exercises three times *each* for 3 days.

2. Use the joint protection methods making a hot drink four times.

3. "Imagine" using the hot drink joint protection methods four times.

4. Take a 2 min break every 30–40 min during work time, resting your hands and arms.

I am sure I can complete this plan (circle):

0   1   2   3   4   5   6   7   8   9   10
(not at all sure)   (totally sure)

When I complete the plan my reward will be:

Tell myself I did a good job! Relax with a mug of hot chocolate.

How well did I do with my plan?

Figure 8.2   Example of an action plan.

3 Initial orientation: Explain why the skill (i.e. joint protection) is performed, its relevance to the person, the objectives of the teaching session and how the person will be participating.
4 Skills teaching: four steps can be used:
   ◦ Demonstrate the whole skill at normal speed *without* commentary, providing a clear image of what is to be learnt. This limits external distraction as the person watches. The therapist must be confident in demonstrating the skill.

- ○ Demonstrate the skill *with* commentary: breaking it down step-by-step. Use clear, *short* instructions. Too much information distracts from motor learning.
- ○ Demonstrate the skill whilst asking the person to provide a commentary: if they are confident in doing so, let them describe each step first before you do it. If not, start/continue each step as a prompt. Errors need correcting, but always allow a few seconds for self-correction first. If not, prompt a re-think or tell the answer if struggling. If in a group, ask the whole group.
- ○ The person demonstrates the skill with commentary. Provide feedback to confirm if correct or prompt them in identifying errors (allowing a few seconds as earlier).

The person thus has multiple chances to watch and hear to aid schema development, before doing it themselves. In a group situation, the last two skills teaching steps can be shared amongst group members (working in pairs or threes; discussing their actions) with each trying the skill in turn. Whilst this may seem lengthy, remember the objective is not just that the person knows what to do, but they develop the psychomotor skills to successfully perform tasks correctly and integrate joint protection into daily life. Repetition facilitates this. Knowing what to do and why does not necessarily lead to behaviour change.

Skills should be gradually developed over three to four treatment sessions, initially starting with blocked practice (i.e. repeating individual tasks such as opening a jar) and progressing rapidly to whole practice (i.e. sequences of activities such as making a hot drink) which progressively require more joint protection methods (e.g. making a meal).

Assessing joint protection education

There are a number of reliable, valid measures for evaluating joint protection education available:

(a) The Joint Protection Knowledge Assessment (Hammond and Lincoln 1999b)
(b) The Joint Protection Self-Efficacy Scale (Niedermann et al. 2010b)
(c) The Joint Protection Behaviour Assessment (Hammond and Lincoln 1999c; Klompenhouwer et al. 2000)

8.11 Practical techniques

A recent study of people with RA ($n = 383$: disease duration 13.2 (SD 10.72) years), using the Evaluation of Daily Activity Questionnaire (Hammond et al. 2011), identified that, of the 120 daily living activities included, 50% or more experienced difficulty in 64 activities; 25–49% in 47; and only 9 activities caused difficulty for fewer than 25% of respondents. Table 8.1 shows some of the most common problems experienced and solutions (Figure 8.3, Figure 8.4, Figure 8.5, Figure 8.6, Figure 8.7 and Figure 8.8).

Table 8.1 Common problems and joint protection solutions.

Common problems	Practical solution
Using a kettle (Figures 8.3 and 8.4)	Heat a cup of water in a microwave. Fill the kettle using a lightweight plastic jug, boil only as much water as is needed. Jug kettle: use two hands, one on the handle, the other firmly pressed against the side (using a cloth) Traditional kettle: two hands on the handle, wrists in extension. If more severe problems: use a kettle tipper.
Open a screw top jar or bottle (Figure 8.5)	Place jar on non-slip mat or damp cloth to avoid slipping and reduce grip strength required from the stabilising hand. Avoid twisting at the fingers by: pressing down using the palm of the hand and turn, with fingers in extension; or using the hand in a cylinder grip, keeping the fingers straight; or use a jar opener, e.g. dycem mat or cone; Baby Boa opener; One Touch Jar Opener.
Opening a tin or a ring-pull can (Figure 8.6)	Use an electric can opener. A variety of ring-pull gadgets are available.
Opening a milk carton	Use a knife to lever up the tab and pierce the aluminium seal.
Plastic bottle	Use a dycem cone jar opener and then a knife to pierce the seal beneath.
Pouring out	Use two hands both firmly in contact with the carton or bottle.
Open a packet/pouch	Use a Slit-a-Pack gadget or Easy-grip scissors.
Slice food (e.g. bread, cheese)	Bread: use an angled bread knife, e.g. Good Grips model Cheese: use a cheese slicer (either a Good Grips or a wire cutter variety, ensuring the handle of the latter is padded).
Carrying a full pan (Figure 8.7)	To reduce the distance carrying a full pan: add the contents to the empty pan when it is on the hob. For example, add water using a plastic jug. Add only the minimum of water needed to reduce weight. Use a flat bottomed ladle to serve straight from the pan to the plates.
Draining water from a pan (e.g. of vegetables, pasta, rice).	Put vegetables into a vegetable (chip) basket. Lift and drain the basket only; wait for the water to cool before emptying the pan. Use a slotted spoon or pasta spoon to drain contents as serving up. Use two hands on the handle, pour the contents into a colander/sieve placed over a bowl in the sink to drain, then rinse contents. Use a steamer to avoid draining.
Peeling and chopping vegetables	Peeling: use an easy grip peeler with a non-slip handle and horizontal blade. Chopping: use a larger, sharper blade, keeping the tip on the board and use point as a pivot; ensure the knife has a larger, non-slip handle to reduce the grip strength required when holding; use frozen vegetables to save chopping.
Turn taps (Figure 8.8)	Use the palm of the hand, fingers straight and press down; use the hand in a cylinder grip, avoid twisting the fingers sideways; use a dycem cone or mat under the palm and turn; use a tap turner; change to lever taps.

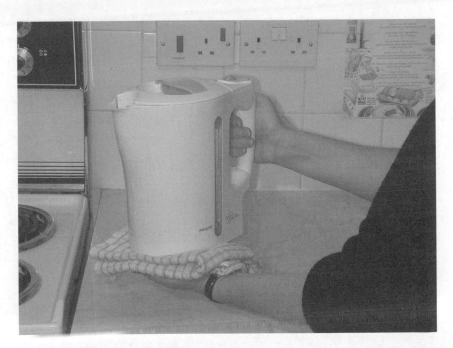

Figure 8.3   Lift kettle: using two hands.

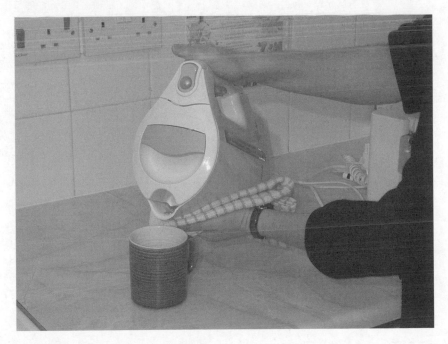

Figure 8.4   Pour kettle: using two hands.

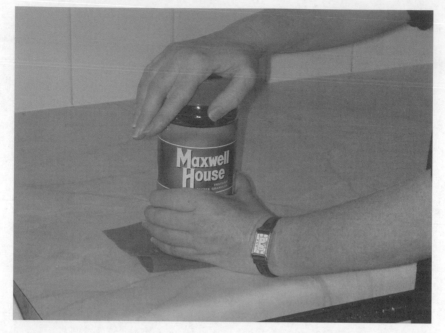

Figure 8.5   Open jar: using palm of hand.

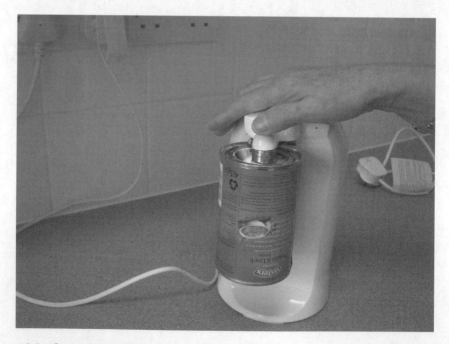

Figure 8.6   Open can: using electric can opener.

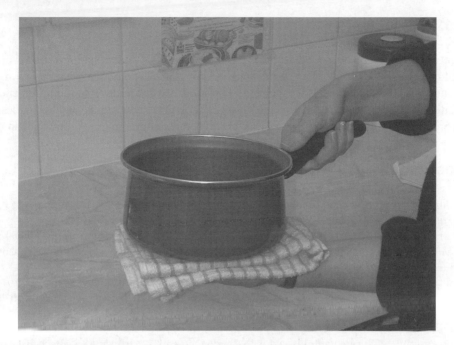

Figure 8.7 Lift pan: using two hands.

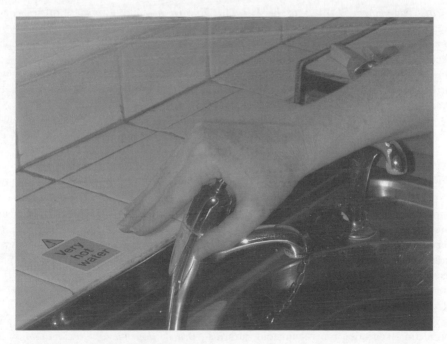

Figure 8.8 Turn tap: using palm of hand.

8.12 Conclusion

Joint protection requires people to change the automatic movement patterns, habits and routines of a lifetime. Providing people with information can help increase motivation to change but rarely major behavioral change. The evidence concludes that joint protection is effective, but only if occupational therapists use cognitive, educational and behavioural techniques, with sufficient supervised practice and home programmes to promote change.

Resources

Arthritis Care (2010) *Independent Living and Arthritis*. http://www.arthritiscare.org.uk/PublicationsandResources/Workindependence. Accessed on 19 March 2012.

Arthritis Research UK (2011a) *Self Help and Daily Living: Looking After Your Joints When You Have Arthritis*. http://www.arthritisresearchuk.org/arthritis-information/arthritis-and-daily-life/looking-after-your-joints.aspx. Accessed on 19 March 2012.

Arthritis Research UK (2011b). *Self Help and Daily Living: Everyday Living and Arthritis*. http://www.arthritisresearchuk.org/arthritis-information/arthritis-and-daily-life/comfort-in-your-home.aspx. Accessed on 19 March 2012.

Arthritis Research UK (2011c) *Self Help and Daily Living: Fatigue*. http://www.arthritisresearchuk.org/arthritis-information/arthritis-and-daily-life/fatigue.aspx. Accessed on 19 March 2012.

Websites

Arthritis Foundation 51 Ways to Be Good to Your Joints. http://www.arthritistoday.org/treatments/self-treatments/joint-health.php. Accessed on 19 March 2012.

Arthritis Foundation Easy to Use Products. http://www.arthritis.org/ease-of-use-new.php. Accessed on 19 March 2012.

Arthritis Society of Canada: Managing Daily Activities: Protecting Your Joints. http://www.arthritis.ca/tips%20for%20living/daily%20activities/default.asp?s=1&province=ca. Accessed on 19 March 2012.

Mayo Clinic, USA. *Rheumatoid Arthritis Pain: Tips for Protecting Your Joints*. http://www.mayoclinic.com/health/arthritis/AR00015. Accessed on 19 March 2012.

References

Adams J, Hammond A, Burridge J, et al. (2005) Static orthoses in the prevention of hand dysfunction in rheumatoid arthritis: A review of the literature. *Musculoskeletal Care* 3(2):85–101.

Arthritis Research UK (2011) *Looking After Your Joints When You Have Arthritis*. http://www.arthritisresearchuk.org/arthritis-information/arthritis-and-daily-life/looking-after-your-joints.aspx. Accessed on 19 March 2012.

Bandura A (1977) Self-efficacy: Towards a unifying theory of behaviour change. *Psychology Reviews* 84:191–215.

Barry MA, Purser J, Hazleman R, et al. (1994) Effect of energy conservation and joint protection education in rheumatoid arthritis. *British Journal of Rheumatology* 33: 1171–1174.

Boustedt C, Nordenskiold U, Lundgren NA (2009) Effects of a hand-joint protection programme with an addition of splinting and exercise: One year follow-up. *Clinical Rheumatology* 28(7):793–799.

Brattstrom M (1987) *Joint Protection and Rehabilitation in Chronic Rheumatic Diseases* (3rd edn.). London: Wolfe Medical.

Buchi S, Sensky T, Sharpe L, et al. (1998) Graphic representation of illness: A novel method of measuring patients' perceptions of the impact of illness. *Psychotherapy and Psychosomatics* 67(4–5):222–225.

Chamberlain MA, Ellis M, Hughes D (1984) Joint protection. *Clinics in the Rheumatic Diseases* 10(3):727–743.

College of Occupational Therapists (2003) *Occupational Therapy Clinical Guidelines for Rheumatology: Joint Protection and Energy Conservation.* London: College of Occupational Therapists.

Cordery JC (1965) Joint protection; a responsibility of the occupational therapist. *American Journal of Occupational Therapists* 19:285–294.

Cordery J, Rocchi M (1998) Joint protection and fatigue management. In: Melvin J, Jensen G. (eds.) *Rheumatologic Rehabilitation. Vol. 1: Assessment and Management.* Bethesda, MD: American Occupational Therapy Association.

Dziedzic K, Hill S, Nicholls E, et al. (2011a) Self management, joint protection education, and exercises in hand osteoarthritis: A randomised controlled trial in the community. *BMC Musculoskeletal Diseases* 12:156.

Dziedzic K, Hill S, Nicholls E, et al. (2011b) Self-management, joint protection and hand exercises in hand osteoarthritis: A multicentred randomised controlled trial in the community. *Annals of the Rheumatic Diseases* 70(Suppl 3):746.

Flatt A (1995) *The Care of the Arthritis Hand* (5th edn.). St Louis, MO: Quality Medical Publishing.

Hammond A (2003) Patient education in arthritis: Helping people change. *Musculoskeletal Care* 1(2):84–97.

Hammond A (2012) *The Lifestyle Management for Arthritis Programme: Leader Manual and Patient Workbooks.* (Available from the author.)

Hammond A (2010) Joint protection and fatigue management. In: Dziedzic KS, Hammond A (eds.) *Rheumatology: Evidence based Practice for Physiotherapists & Occupational Therapists.* Edinburgh, UK: Churchill Livingstone Elsevier.

Hammond A, Freeman K (2001) One year outcomes of a randomised controlled trial of an educational-behavioural joint protection programme for people with rheumatoid arthritis. *Rheumatology* 40:1044–1051.

Hammond A, Freeman K (2004) The long term outcomes from a randomised controlled trial of an educational-behavioural joint protection programme for people with rheumatoid arthritis. *Clinical Rehabilitation* 18:520–528.

Hammond A, Lincoln N (1999a) Effect of a joint protection programme for people with rheumatoid arthritis. *Clinical Rehabilitation* 13:392–400.

Hammond A, Lincoln N (1999b) The Joint Protection Knowledge Assessment: Reliability and validity. *British Journal of Occupational Therapy* 62(3):117–122.

Hammond A, Lincoln N (1999c) Development of the Joint Protection Behaviour Assessment. *Arthritis Care and Research* 12(3):200–207.

Hammond A, Niedermann K (2010) Patient education and self management. In: Dziedzic KS, Hammond A (eds.) *Rheumatology: Evidence based Practice for Physiotherapists & Occupational Therapists.* Edinburgh, UK: Churchill Livingstone Elsevier.

Hammond A, Lincoln N, Sutcliffe L (1999) A crossover trial evaluating an educational-behavioural joint protection programme for people with rheumatoid arthritis. *Patient Education and Counselling* 37:19–32.

Hammond A, Bryan J, Hardy A (2008) Effects of a modular behavioural arthritis education programme: A pragmatic parallel group randomized controlled trial. *Rheumatology* 47(11):1712–1718.

Hammond A, Tennant A, Tyson S, et al. (2011) Development of the United Kingdom evaluation of daily activities questionnaire in rheumatoid arthritis using Rasch Analysis. *Arthritis & Rheumatism* 63(10 Suppl 1000):2555.

Iversen M, Hammond A, Betteridge N (2010) Self-management of rheumatic diseases: State of the art and future directions. *Annals of the Rheumatic Diseases* 69:955–963.

Klompenhouwer P, Lysack C, Dijkers M, et al. (2000) The joint protection behaviour assessment: A reliability study. *American Journal of Occupational Therapy* 54(5):516–524.

Lorig K, Holman H, Sobel D, et al. (2007) Becoming an active self-manager. In: *Living a Healthy Life with Chronic Conditions: Self-Management of Heart Disease, Arthritis, Diabetes, Asthma, Bronchitis, Emphysema and Others* (3rd edn., pp. 17–31). Palo Alto, CA: Bull Publishing Company.

Mackway-Jones K, Walker M (1999) *Pocket Guide to Teaching for Medical Instructors*. London: BMJ Books.

Masiero S, Boniolo A, Wassermann L, et al. (2007) Effects of an educational-behavioural joint protection program on people with moderate to severe rheumatoid arthritis: A randomized controlled trial. *Clinical Rheumatology* 26:2043–2050.

Mason P, Butler C (2010) Assessing importance, confidence and readiness. In: *Health Behaviour Change: A Guide for Practitioners* (2nd edn., pp. 55–70). Edinburgh, UK: Churchill Livingstone.

Melvin JL (1989) *Rheumatic Disease in the Adult and Child: Occupational Therapy and Rehabilitation* (3rd edn.). Philadelphia, PA: FA Davis.

Niedermann K, Hammond A, Forster A, et al. (2010a) Perceived benefits and barriers to join protection among people with rheumatoid arthritis and occupational therapists: A mixed methods study. *Musculoskeletal Care* 8:143–156.

Niedermann K, Forster A, Ciurea A, et al. (2010b) Development and psychometric properties of a joint protection self-efficacy scale. *Scandinavian Journal of Occupational Therapy* 18(2):143–152.

Niedermann K, de Bie RA, Kubli R, et al. (2011) Effectiveness of individual resource-oriented joint protection education in people with rheumatoid arthritis. A randomized controlled trial. *Patient Education & Counseling* 82(1):42–48.

Prochaska JO, DiClemente CC (1992) Stages of change in the modification of problem behaviours. In: Hersen M, Eisler RM, Miller PM (eds.) *Progress in Behaviour Modification*. Champaign, IL: Sycamore Press.

Schmidt R, Lee T (2005) *Motor Control and Learning: A Behavioural Emphasis* (4th edn.). Champaign, IL: Human Kinetics Europe Ltd.

Sheon RP (1985) A joint protection guide for non-articular rheumatic disorders. *Postgraduate Medicine* 77:329–337.

Stamm T, Machold KP, Smolen JS (2002) Joint protection and home hand exercises improve hand function in patients with hand osteoarthritis: A randomized controlled trial. *Arthritis Care and Research* 47:44–49.

Ward V, Hill J, Hale C, et al. (2007) Patient priorities of care in rheumatology out-patient clinics: A qualitative study. *Musculoskeletal Care* 5(4):216–228.

Chapter 9

Pain management

Lucy Reeve[1] and Margaret McArthur[2]

[1]*Rheumatology Department, Norfolk and Norwich Univesity Hospital, Norfolk, United Kingdom;*
[2]*School of Allied Health Professions, University of East Anglia, Norfolk, United Kingdom*

9.1 Introduction

> It is easier to find men who will volunteer to die, than to find those who are willing to endure pain with patience. (Julius Caesar)

Pain is surely the most common reason that people seek medical attention and this is particularly evident in the field of rheumatology (Montecucco et al. 2009). In fact pain is frequently the first symptom in the majority of rheumatic conditions, generally resulting in a significant burden of suffering, deeply affecting clients' quality of life (NICE 2009, p. 7; WHO 2003) and also influencing the lifestyle of families involved (Locker 1983; Main and Williams 2002). Moreover, the burden of rheumatic pain is also economic, with a large amount of direct (e.g. drugs, medical care) and indirect costs (e.g. work disability) (Montecucco et al. 2009).

9.2 What is pain?

> Pain is an unpleasant sensory and emotional experience associated with actual or potential tissue damage or described in terms of such damage. (IASP 2011)

Pain is a multifactorial sensation involving peripheral nociception, central sensitisation and cortical interpretation (Katz and Rottenberg 2005). Generally pain is categorised as nociceptive when arising in areas of tissue damage and neurogenic when associated with specific nerve damage. 'Nociceptors' are special neurones in the tissues that respond to all manner of stimuli *if* those stimuli are sufficient to be potentially

Rheumatology Practice in Occupational Therapy: Promoting Lifestyle Management, First Edition.
Edited by Lynne Goodacre and Margaret McArthur.
© 2013 John Wiley & Sons, Ltd. Published 2013 by John Wiley & Sons, Ltd.

damaging to the tissue. 'Nociception' involves the stimulation of nerves that convey information about potential tissue damage to the brain and is the most common, but by no means the only, precursor to pain (Butler and Moseley 2003).

The mechanisms of pain perception are complex, involving extensive neurobiology and affective, cognitive and behavioural factors. So, the relationship between pain and tissue injury or damage and disease is never straightforward (Kojima et al. 2009; Wall 1999), as people may experience similar levels of pain independently from the underlying pathological condition (Sheane et al. 2008). Pain is a subjective experience involving a complex interplay of sensory, emotional and physical factors, which involve many parts of the peripheral and central nervous system (Mann and Carr 2009). The *actual* pain that is experienced is a subjective perception that results from the transduction, transmission and modulation of many forms of sensory information. This sensory input may be filtered through a person's genetic composition, prior learning history, current psychological status and socio-cultural influences (Gatchel et al. 2007).

Pain is never an isolated sensation; it is always accompanied by emotion and meaning (Wall 1999). Emotion is an immediate reaction to nociception (or other aversive events associated with it), which is followed by a cognitive response where the brain attaches meaning to the emotional experience and may trigger additional emotional reactions and amplify the experience of pain, thus perpetuating a vicious circle of nociception, pain, distress and disability (Gatchel et al. 2007).

Whatever the cause of pain, the effect tends to be pervasive, influencing the person's mood, personality and social relationships. Depression, sleep disturbance, fatigue and decreased overall physical and mental functioning are common experiences. As a result, pain is only one of many issues that must be addressed in the management of ongoing pain. Single interventions that only tackle the biomedical source of pain, without addressing psychological and social stresses, are unlikely to be effective in the long term (Ashburn and Staats 1999).

9.3   Pain and rheumatology

There are several types of pain associated with rheumatic conditions, including inflammatory (e.g. joint synovitis), biomechanical (e.g. joint damage) and neuropathic pain (e.g. carpal tunnel syndrome) (Montecucco et al. 2009). Rheumatic conditions are typically associated with chronic pain, and pain control is not always easily achievable, thus representing a very important problem for both client and clinician (Sheane et al. 2008).

Inflammation evokes complex changes in the peripheral and central nervous system, leading to a state of hyperalgesia (enhanced pain during noxious stimulation) and allodynia (pain from innocuous stimuli, e.g. gentle pressure and movement) and consequently persistent pain. In ongoing chronic disease, intense continuing stimulation of nociceptors, such as that seen with prolonged and significant joint inflammation or mechanical damage, causes long-term changes in noxious transmission leading to structural and functional changes within the central nervous systems. For some people, these changes mean that pain can continue despite subsequent resolution of inflammation. This is called central sensitisation or Wind Up (Parsons and Preece 2010; Wall 1999). Changes in the nervous system may also lead to neuropathic pain, which is most commonly due to nerve entrapment, e.g. carpal tunnel syndrome (Rosenbaum 2001).

In addition, there is pain typical of fibromyalgia, a syndrome of unclear pathogenesis, characterised by long-lasting, widespread musculoskeletal pain. This presents with a reduced threshold for pain in the muscles, together with many other non-musculoskeletal symptoms including fatigue, sleep disturbance, headache and variable bowel habits (Bliddal 2007). Therefore, therapists need a working knowledge of the pathophysiology of rheumatic conditions and potential causes of pain so that they can educate clients about the different types of pain they may experience and the best way to manage these. For example, it is important that people can distinguish between what is a normal background level of pain and what is pain associated with acute inflammation, because these need to be treated differently, both medically and behaviourally (Sandles 1990).

9.4 Living with rheumatic pain

For those with rheumatic conditions, the experience of pain is surrounded by uncertainty. The pain varies in intensity, duration and location in the person's body. It is also unpredictable, meaning that people can never accurately forecast how they are going to be. These characteristics of variability and unpredictability make the pain itself more difficult to manage and exacerbate the disruptive effect of pain on a person's life. For example, pain may be present in one joint one day and another the next, so the kinds of activities they are able to do are constantly changing and the nature of the difficulty they have with a given task will also change. Consequently, coping on a daily basis requires a wide repertoire of strategies in order to deal with ever-changing circumstances and means that forward planning is almost impossible. People need to be flexible and lower their expectations to deal with this and constantly reappraise and alter their daily activities (Persson et al. 2011; Wiener 1975).

As well as being unable to predict when levels of pain will increase or flare ups will occur, people often cannot explain why this should happen. Even day-to-day variation may be something of a mystery, which leads people to constantly try and find suitable explanations that made sense to them (Locker 1983). Not surprisingly constant self-monitoring and hypervigilance for pain can develop (Mengshoel 2008; Vroman et al. 2009). Unfortunately, pain is an ambiguous indicator of the course of the disease. Sudden increases or decreases in pain could be read as nothing more than the normal variation of pain levels or taken to be an indicator of a longer-term improvement or decline in their condition. Furthermore, this typical pattern of variation and unpredictability may also mean that certain pain management strategies are not always successful (Locker 1983). What 'works', i.e. what controls pain and inflammation one day, or week, may not work the next (Wiener 1975).

9.5   Pain assessment

The biopsychosocial model is a widely accepted and heuristic perspective to the understanding and treatment of chronic pain (Gatchel et al. 2007) and is an approach that occupational therapists have used in their pain assessment for many years (Milne 1983). This understanding and approach to treatment is particularly important because pain is not a single measurable response like blood pressure or pulse; for the person in pain, it is a total experience that cannot be objectively measured (Mann and Carr 2009). Therefore, the assessment of pain is much more than just obtaining a measurement of pain levels or location; it is the starting point of the package of care.

The initial interview is a crucial stage in the pain management process because it permits an in-depth exploration of someone's experience from their unique perspective. Most importantly, it provides people with an opportunity to express their pain and tell their story. When the therapist actively listens and conveys genuine interest in their pain, it helps to build a therapeutic relationship and gives people an active role in their own pain management (Mann and Carr 2009; Strong et al. 2002). Many studies have explored the experiences of people with chronic pain and found that the most important factor for clients was that their pain was believed and their distress acknowledged (Mann and Carr 2009; Seers and Friedli 1996). Therefore, it is important to dedicate ample time to this process rather than moving quickly to action, e.g. providing an orthosis or behavioural advice (Vroman et al. 2009).

There is extensive literature about the measurement of the pain experience, with many measurements available and many more being developed, thereby making the selection of an appropriate tool a difficult task (Parsons and Preece 2010). Strong et al. (2002) suggest there are three components that need to be considered. These include:

- a description of the pain (e.g. location, severity and type of sensation),
- responses to the pain (e.g. changes in behaviours, fears, attitudes, beliefs and confidence) and
- impact of pain on a person's life (e.g. functional status and levels of activity).

Clinically, one of the most effective models for the assessment and treatment of pain is based on the Cognitive Behavioural Therapy Model (CBTM) (Cole et al. 2005; David 2006, 2010). The CBTM provides a simple structured method where the therapist asks questions about the five areas of life shown in Figure 9.1: Thoughts, Feelings, Physical Symptoms, Behaviours and Environmental Factors (Cole et al 2005; Greenberger and Padesky 1995).

This dynamic model addresses five aspects of life that are interconnected and constantly influencing all the others. Ongoing pain can have a profound impact on all areas. For example: thoughts (I *should* be able to do all the activities I used to do), feelings (sadness), behaviours (I *must* keep going until I complete the activity) and symptoms (increased pain/inflammation/fatigue). Lastly, questions about environmental factors provide information on the personal circumstances of each individual such as their roles and responsibilities, levels of social support and the physical environment in which they operate (Figure 9.2).

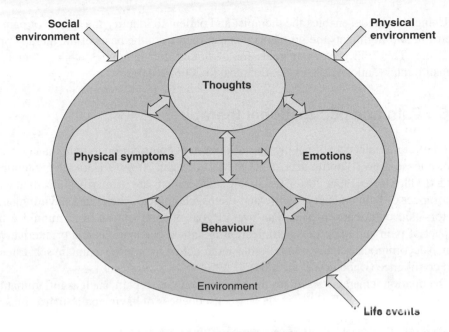

Figure 9.1 The Cognitive Behavioural Therapy Model (CBTM).

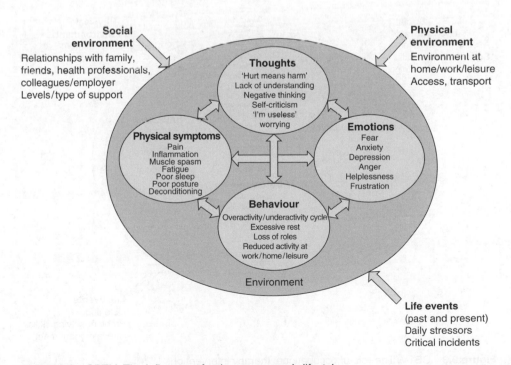

Figure 9.2 CBTM. The influence of pain on a person's lifestyle.

Using this model enables the therapist and patient to identify the effects of pain in their life *and* highlights the problems that can then form the basis of the therapy programme. This will give clear goals for treatment and outcomes against which to measure intervention (Cole et al. 2005; David 2006, 2010).

9.6 Pain and occupational therapy

The literature on occupational therapists' important contribution to pain management continues to grow (Hammond et al. 2008; Macedo et al. 2009; O'Hara 1996; Steutjens et al. 2008; Strong 1996, 2002). Occupational therapists are primarily concerned with the impact of pain on everyday life and the psychological, social and environmental factors that contribute to pain. The overall goal of intervention is to minimise the impact of pain and maximise participation in valued occupations and/or alternatives which accommodate changes in self, role and function in order to maintain self-esteem and confidence (Dubouloz et al. 2004).

Occupational therapists address the primary sources of pain, such as inflammation or joint damage, as well as the secondary consequences of having pain such as muscle spasm, poor sleep, physical deconditioning and fatigue. Interventions include client education; changing behaviour (see Chapter 7), including joint protection education (see Chapter 8); correct body positioning, postural advice and manual handling techniques; environmental adaptation and use of assistive equipment (see Chapter 10);

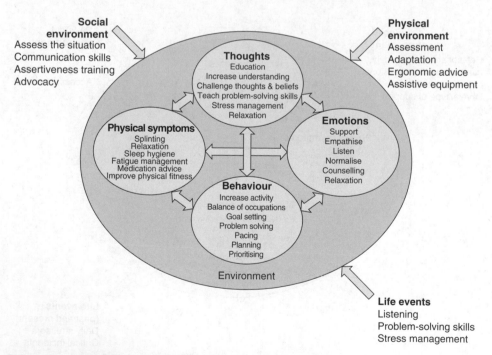

Figure 9.3 CBTM. The role of occupational therapy interventions.

provision of orthoses (see Chapter 12); vocational rehabilitation (see Chapter 11); and counselling and stress management, relaxation and sleep hygiene (Hammond et al. 2008). Figure 9.3 shows how these interventions fit into the five areas of the CBTM.

9.7   Patient education

From diagnosis onwards, people with rheumatic conditions require the necessary knowledge, understanding, skills and confidence to make informed decisions concerning treatment options, to follow treatment regimes and perform self-care activities (Barlow 2009).

There are many myths, misunderstandings and unnecessary fears about pain. Patients' beliefs about the cause or meaning of their pain will contribute to how they experience their pain and how much pain impacts upon their daily life. Therefore, in order for treatment to be effective, client education must not simply fill gaps in knowledge but build on the client's already held beliefs, attitudes and behaviours (Kett et al. 2010). Pain is most effectively controlled when it is understood. Anxiety is commonly associated with pain. People worry about the 'meaning' of the pain, why it is there, what is causing it and what is going on. They also worry about the future and how the pain will affect them, and the impact it will have on their lives. Fear generates anxiety, and anxiety focuses the attention. The more attention is locked, the worse the pain is (Gatchel et al. 2007; Wall 1999).

People who understand the causes, significance and aggravating factors of their pain are much more likely to be able to manage it (Shlotzhauer and McGuire 2003). Asking questions to elicit clients' current understanding, beliefs and thoughts about their pain is a useful starting point to pain management.

9.8   Fatigue management

For many people, fatigue can be the most incapacitating feature of having a rheumatic disease (Hewlett et al. 2010; Minnock and Bresnihan 2004). Like pain, fatigue is unpredictable and can significantly impact on all aspects of a person's life (NRAS 2010). Fatigue is a multidimensional symptom that is experienced physically, cognitively and emotionally. Physical manifestations include decreased strength and endurance; cognitive fatigue contributes to forgetfulness, diminished concentration, decreased attention span and/or lack of motivation; and emotional responses range from anger and frustration to anxiety and depression.

Fatigue is not always proportionate to exertion or activity level; it can occur continuously, appear intermittently and exacerbate other symptoms, especially pain. Although the mechanisms that lead to fatigue are not completely understood, several variables, singly or in combination, may contribute. For example, fatigue is associated with disease processes such as inflammation or anaemia, as well as being a consequence of de-conditioning, poor sleep that is disturbed by pain and emotional reactions, such as depression (Hewlett et al. 2010).

There is a close correlation between pain and fatigue. People who experience fatigue are known to be at more risk of pain (and vice versa) (NICE 2009; Riemsma et al. 1998). Therefore, strategies designed to manage fatigue may also have a beneficial effect on pain. People with fatigue are faced with daily decisions about how they should spend their energy so they can continue to participate in activities that are meaningful to them and make the most out of the energy. Fortuitously, many of the pain management strategies discussed in this chapter can also be effective for fatigue (Furst et al. 1987).

9.9   Sleep hygiene

Many people with pain have difficulties with sleeping (Cole et al. 2005; Taylor-Gjevre et al. 2011). Pain often causes disturbance in sleeping patterns, interferes with the ability to initiate sleep and impairs the quality and duration of sleep. Once again, this is a reciprocal relationship where poor sleep then *causes* increased pain and disability (Hughes 2009), increased fatigue and irritability (Lamberg 1999) and psychological disturbance (Strong 2002). Therefore, therapists need to consistently enquire about sleep and use suitable behavioural and cognitive strategies as part of the treatment programme to improve it. Interventions may include modification of sleep patterns and the sleep environment, use of relaxation and stress management techniques, effective use of medication and appropriate positioning (Keable 1997; Strong 1996, 2002).

9.10   Medication

Some peoples' symptoms are greatly improved and pain practically eliminated for extended periods of time by the effectiveness of medication. The pharmacological management of pain is a complex area. Drug therapies provide an important means of managing pain. In rheumatological practice, there are a number of different groups of drugs that produce pain relief through a variety of mechanisms, with varying degrees of effectiveness (Parsons and Preece 2010). Unfortunately, fear and distrust in medication and poor adherence to treatment may contribute to sub-optimal pain control (Montecucco et al. 2009).

Having knowledge of the actions and side effects of such medications enables therapists to be proactive in advocating for effective management of clients' pain. This is especially advantageous where effective pain control would enhance compliance with other aspects of their therapy and permit engagement in daily activities (Wright et al. 2002).

9.11   Changing behaviour

Pain has a profound effect on participation in everyday activities at home, work and leisure, leading to the development of an increasingly sedentary and unfulfilling lifestyle which can have an impact on fitness and mood (Penny et al. 1999; Skevington

1998; Strong 1996). Many people reduce their participation in activities to prevent increases in pain, e.g. avoiding certain behaviour or movements that are associated with an escalation in pain or thought to cause damage. Reducing activity is a common sense response to pain, and it is not surprising that people try their best to rest or avoid activities that make pain worse. Other people attempt to 'carry on regardless', driven by the notion of 'not wanting to give in to pain' until a severe episode of pain or exhaustion necessitates a break. This leads to the development of an overactivity–underactivity cycle where periods of excessive activity alternate with prolonged rest (David 2006, 2010; O'Hara 1996). Fear of exacerbating pain also leads some people to perform activities in a tense, careful way leading to excessive muscle tension, which can further increase pain (Birkholtz et al. 2004).

As a result of pain, people are forced to pay attention to the performance of activities and figure out new or altered ways of carrying them out (Alsaker et al. 2009). Pain may be reduced or relieved by altering the methods normally used to complete an activity, adjusting a person's lifestyle or adopting a new pattern of behaviour (David 2006, 2010). Using their skills of activity analysis, occupational therapists work with people to identify how pain is problematic in their daily lives, such as what it prevents them doing, and create an intervention plan that will provide the support and skills people need for continued participation and engagement in valued roles.

Pacing

Pacing is an overarching strategy that is recommended as an effective way of carrying out activities to reduce pain (and fatigue). Various strategies are described under the heading of pacing. For example, achieving a balance between activity and rest; changing position and activity; taking frequent short rests; breaking tasks into manageable bits and alternating positions and tasks frequently. Pacing also involves careful planning and prioritisation of a person's activities, delegation of tasks (or elements of tasks to others); adopting a creative, flexible problem-solving approach to activities to deal with constantly changing symptoms and ensuring that goals are realistic and achievable (Birkholtz et al. 2004; O'Hara 1996; Strong 2002; Vaughn et al. 2008).

Goal setting is an inherent part of the pacing process. People are encouraged to set realistic baselines for activities, which are achievable on both 'good' and 'bad' days. These are then increased gradually, in accordance with the steps identified in the goal-setting process, rather than being led by pain levels, where a person does as much as they feel able to do according to how they feel at the time (Cole et al. 2005; O'Hara 1996). The use of timers has been described as a beneficial addition to this process, ensuring that people are prompted to change position or activity according to time, rather than pain (Birkholtz et al. 2004).

During a 'flare up' of pain (and or inflammation), the person reduces activity back to baseline, rather than complete rest, and then returns to building up activities once things have improved (O'Hara 1996). Effective pacing not only helps with pain management but enables someone to build physical strength and stamina, and develop confidence in their abilities. When it comes to taking action and achieving goals, a large part of the success is related to our mindset and the beliefs we hold about ourselves. For example, people may be motivated to increase activity, but on the other hand they may perceive activity to be uncomfortable and be anxious that it might aggravate their pain.

People need to believe that they can change and have the confidence to take action. Taking small steps builds self-efficacy, which increases motivation and confidence to take further steps. Research indicates that people achieve more when they work towards rheumatic conditions-specific, challenging, but achievable goals that have deadlines and reward rheumatic conditions associated with them (Yeung 2010). Writing down goals increases the likelihood they will be achieved, as does identification of any potential obstacles and strategies that can be used to overcome them (Greenberger and Padesky 1995). Goal setting is enhanced by teaching people to use a problem-solving approach. Problem-focused strategies involve defining the problem, generating alternative solutions, weighing up the costs and benefits of each alternative and then taking action (Cole et al. 2005). People are encouraged to step back from their usual routines and think about how they can do things differently; using 'behavioural experiments' to discover what really happens when they do something, rather than what they *think* will happen (Greenberger and Padesky 1995).

Learning new ways of functioning in daily life is a central challenge for people with rheumatic conditions which necessitate a process of personal change (Vaughn et al. 2008). Whilst the objective of therapists is to support clients in fulfilling their different occupational roles by modification of their behaviour, unfortunately this is often accepted with difficulty and not maintained over time because these interventions conflict with peoples' existing beliefs. For example, asking for help may be perceived as 'giving in' by conflicting with a personal value of independence and lead people to think that they were 'useless' and 'incapacitated'. Alternatively, if a person believes that it is 'important to finish what they start' or sees rest as a 'waste of time' believing that to 'do less is lazy', then the use of pacing strategies may induce feelings of guilt (Dubouloz et al. 2008). The fluctuating nature of pain (and fatigue) does not facilitate change because it maintains hope for improvement without the need to change their way of doing things (Locker 1983). Therefore, to encourage behavioural change, therapists need to recognise and address these beliefs and present these principles in a way that is meaningful to each individual (Dubouloz et al. 2008).

9.12   Vocational rehabilitation

Pain has a significant impact on peoples' ability to work. Vocational rehabilitation is an area where occupational therapists have particular expertise, and this is discussed (Gilworth et al. 2001) in detail in Chapter 11. However, it is evident that all the interventions associated with pain management described in this chapter should be extended into the workplace in order to reduce pain and increase a person's independence or ability (Melvin and Jensen 2000).

9.13 Psychological interventions

Pain severity has a strong relationship with psychological well-being (Gatchel et al. 2007). Psychological distress has been shown to have an impact on pain perception in systemic lupus erythematosus, rheumatoid arthritis (RA) and fibromyalgia (Arthritis Care 2011; Montecucco et al. 2009). Psychological factors modulate the experience of pain and can predispose people to experience more pain. Coping with pain and illness provokes a range of responses including fear, frustration, anxiety, confusion, uncertainty, loss, despair and depression. These responses are experienced as the person attempts to process and adjust to the consequent impact on their lives and those around them (McKenna 2007).

High levels of anxiety and depression have been shown to be associated with pain, with observational studies showing that pain, lack of control over pain and dissatisfaction with abilities affected psychological well-being, self-esteem and adjustment to disease (NICE 2009). However, given its persistent and pervasive nature, it is not surprising that pain has been identified as a correlate of depression in RA (Creed and Ash 1992; Dickens et al. 2002), osteoarthritis (Summers et al. 1988) and ankylosing spondylitis (Barlow 2009), with pain (and fatigue) being the best overall predictors of self-reported depression (Wolfe and Michaud 2009).

The relationship between psychosocial problems and pain is complex and bidirectional, with both factors influencing each other (MacKichan et al. 2008). Depression is associated with greater pain intensity and unpleasantness, more bodily sites of pain and a higher degree of pain-related disability. Furthermore, there is potential overlap between the symptoms of rheumatic conditions and depression, as depression in itself is *also* associated with a loss of valued activities, social isolation fatigue and sleep disturbance (Katz and Yelin 2001). Interestingly, inflammatory mediators have also been linked to the pathophysiology of depression (Elenkov 2008), meaning that depression may be a primary symptom of rheumatic conditions as well as a secondary effect.

In addition, there appears to be evidence of linkages between stressful events and more severe pain, with variables such as social support acting as a buffer (Affleck et al. 1987, 1994). Many people mention physical and emotional stress as a cause of additional pain and try as far as possible to avoid a situation where this is likely. Daily stressors and life events can provoke emotional reactions which cause physiological arousal, with accompanying muscle tension, poor sleep and fatigue. All these factors feed into the vicious cycle of pain which is difficult to break (Shlotzhauer and McGuire 2003). Of course, having a chronic illness magnifies the stresses of everyday life and creates new stresses. The onset of a chronic disease can pose a considerable threat to self-concept and lead to varying degrees of stress and anxiety (Bury 1991). Uncertainty is perhaps the most stressful aspect of life. Unfortunately, uncertainty and unpredictability are inherent characteristics of rheumatic pain (and fatigue) which change from one day to the next, or even within the same day, making even short-term planning fraught with worry and anxiety (Locker 1983).

Psychological distress can often be overlooked in clinical settings where the primary focus is on the physical aspects of the condition (Barlow 2009). It is often the occupational therapist who identifies psychological issues and provides the necessary counselling and support to deal with the psychological distress associated with pain (and fatigue), which are such an essential part of the overall pain management strategy. The importance of a person-centred approach (Cole et al. 2005; Rogers 1959) including active listening, empathetic understanding of the pain experience and most importantly acknowledgement of someone's distress has already been highlighted in the section on pain assessment. Overall, it is clear that addressing underlying psychological distress is an essential element of any pain management plan and demonstrates the potential for therapists to improve pain control by addressing their clients' psychological symptoms. This is supported by the literature which indicates that psychological interventions commonly provided by occupational therapists, such as counselling, stress management, use of CBT, relaxation and teaching cognitive coping skills, significantly reduce pain and improve functional ability and psychological status (Astin et al. 2002; Backman 2006).

Cognitive behavioural therapy

Other psychological approaches to managing pain, such as CBT, are designed to alter the psychological processes that can significantly contribute to pain, distress and disability (David 2006, 2010). CBT is a practical psychological therapy that can help people with ongoing pain. The goal is to help people change any negative thoughts and unhelpful behaviours which increase pain, disability and emotional distress and negatively influence all aspects of a person's life (Evers et al. 2002). It is a particularly appropriate approach for occupational therapists due to its collaborative, structured and goal-orientated approach, and the fact that it involves teaching clients to take control of their pain by giving them the skills to overcome problems using a problem-solving approach (Beck 2006; David 2006, 2010).

Stress management

Stress management techniques are also commonly used by occupational therapists working with people with pain (Hammond et al. 2008; Macedo et al. 2009; O'Hara 1996; Strong 1996). Stress management can be useful in enabling people to identify particular stressors in their lives, learn about the body's response to stress and the impact this has on their pain (fatigue and mood). Various strategies may be introduced dependent on the nature of the stressors involved including relaxation, assertiveness training, communication skills, problem solving and goal setting (Macedo et al. 2009; O'Hara 1996; Strong 1996).

Encouraging occupational balance may also contribute to psychological well-being as it seems many people eliminate leisure activities to leave more energy for work and basic activities of daily living. However, given that participation in meaningful leisure activities is more closely linked to well-being than participation in other occupations, this may negatively influence their quality of life (Locker 1983; Skjutar et al. 2010;

Stout and Finlayson 2011). Enjoyable activities also seem to provide an excellent way of distracting someone from their pain by taking the mind away from the internal experience of pain and enabling them to become engrossed on the task in hand (Persson et al. 2011).

Relaxation

Relaxation techniques are commonly used by occupational therapists for pain management (Hammond et al. 2008; O'Hara 1996; Strong 1996, 2002). They can be classed as primarily physical or mental (Payne 2000). Physical techniques, such as Mitchell's simple relaxation, progressive muscular relaxation, passive relaxation and breathing methods, are predominantly aimed at reducing the pain associated with local muscle spasm around affected joints, whereas mental techniques such as guided imagery, visualisation and meditation may have a positive effect on the general physiological arousal that is associated with the stress response, anxiety and depression precipitated by the effects of having a chronic illness and ongoing pain (Keable 1997; Strong 2002). It is also thought that relaxation has an impact on pain by promoting the release of endorphins, endogenous neuropeptides, which are associated with a sense of well-being and pain suppression, and/or cognitive distraction, i.e. diverting attention away from the pain (Keable 1997; Wall 1999; Wells and Nown 1993). However, pain management may not always be the primary goal of relaxation; relaxation may be aimed at stress management or improvement of sleep, although reduction of pain may occur as a secondary effect if these problems are more effectively managed (Cole et al. 2005).

In rheumatic conditions where pain is multifaceted, combinations of different relaxation techniques may be more effective than a single technique (Keable 1997). Unfortunately, the literature regarding the use of relaxation in the management of rheumatic pain provides little clarity about the exact mechanism by which it works, or which is the most effective relaxation technique to use (Carroll and Seers 1998). Some studies suggest that imaginative reinterpretation of the pain and replacing pain words with expressions like 'a certain feeling' are more useful than techniques that focus on attention diversion (e.g. guided imagery). Guided imagery for pain relief is a popular relaxation technique, and studies indicate that using pleasant or neutral imagery is more effective than pain acknowledgement for relieving pain (Newman et al. 1996).

Regardless of the relaxation technique used, relaxation is a skill to be learnt, which is most effective when used on a regular basis so people should be encouraged to find ways to integrate relaxation into their daily life routines to increase the likelihood it will continue to be used (Keable 1997; Payne 2000; Strong 2002). However, relaxation is not a strategy that everyone finds helpful. Some people do not enjoy relaxing; others find that focusing on the body intensifies their perception of pain, and those with acute joint inflammation are not advised to use tense release methods (e.g. progressive muscular relaxation). Furthermore, there are certain comorbidities such as certain psychiatric and cardiac conditions where relaxation may not be advised (Payne 2000). Luckily, there are countless other means by which someone may achieve relaxation; a long bath combined with relaxing music, a gentle massage or just relaxing your mind by engaging in an enjoyable task or talking to a friend can reduce emotional and physical tension (Shlotzhauer and McGuire 2003). Ideally therapists should have a repertoire of techniques which can be tailored to the specific condition and needs of each individual.

Mindfulness

Lastly, there is growing interest in the clinical application of mindfulness meditation. Mindfulness is an integral part of acceptance-based approaches to pain management which are intended to produce positive physical and psychosocial adjustment, by enabling people to live with things that cannot be changed, such as pain and disability (Cole et al. 2005; McCracken and Vowles 2006). Mindfulness has origins in Eastern meditation traditions, but has been incorporated into clinical interventions (Baer 2005). Mindfulness training has been shown to provide lasting improvements in psychological well-being and pain-related coping in people with rheumatic conditions (Grossman 2007; Hawtin and Sullivan 2011; Pradhan 2007) and is especially beneficial for those with chronic depression (Zautra et al. 2008). Mindfulness is not a relaxation exercise but may produce a relaxed state or improve mood (Germer 2005). It may also reduce stress responses, increase awareness of negative thinking and increase self-acceptance, and have physical benefits such as improving posture, sleep and breathing; reducing pain and enabling people to listen to their body (Thompson 2009), all of which are therapeutic goals in the management of rheumatic pain.

9.14   Social support

Chronic illness and pain disrupts family life and invariably causes changes in family roles and circumstances. In one study of clients with RA, pain was identified as the most frequent source of family problems, with people stating that their pain made them irritable and bad tempered in ways that constantly threatened to affect family relationships (Locker 1983).

   Pain is a private invisible experience. This invisibility, coupled with the unpredictability of pain, often makes it difficult for significant others to understand the sufferer's experience and distress (Arthritis Care 2011; Vroman et al. 2009). Interpersonal difficulties with significant others, including partners, health professionals and employers, are common (Strong 1996). People often report that those around them still have the same expectations of them prior to disease onset and find it hard to really understand their experiences (Barlow 2009; Vaughn et al. 2008). Problematic support (such as lack of sympathy or understanding from social networks) has been associated with higher levels of pain (and fatigue) among people with RA (Locker 1983; Riemsma et al. 1998). Unfortunately, although maintaining a social network of friends and family that provides appropriate positive support contributes to psychological well-being, it appears that the presence of ongoing pain leads to reduced social engagement (Hughes 2009; Locker 1983; Stamm et al. 2004).

Partnerships are also threatened in other ways by ongoing pain, most notably because of the adverse effects on sexual interest and activity (Locker 1983; NRAS 2004; Reisine et al. 1987; Strong 2002). Fears that sex will increase pain and partners' fears that they will hurt the person are common (NRAS 2004). However, sexual problems can be managed in the same way as other daily activities and be eased by pacing sexual activities, challenging unhelpful thoughts and feelings and by experimenting to find comfortable positions for sexual intercourse (Cole et al. 2005).

So, it is clear that gaining an understanding about the nature of relationships with family, friends, work colleagues and employers is essential in establishing the types of support available and the influence this may be having on a person's pain and health in general. Assertiveness and communication skills training may be particularly beneficial to enable someone to deal with the interpersonal difficulties they may be experiencing as a consequence of their pain, along with counselling and support where this is absent in their own environment (Cole et al. 2005; Strong 1996).

9.15 Summary

People living with rheumatic pain constitute an important target group for all health professionals; but given the disruption pain causes within an individual's life, it would seem clear that the occupational therapist is central to the pain management process. Pain management is a complex and challenging area, as clients are at increased risk of emotional disorders (anxiety and depression), maladaptive thinking (catastrophising and worrying), functional deficits and physical de-conditioning. All of these variables are interrelated and cannot be treated in isolation. Occupational therapy education in both physical and mental health and their holistic approach to assessment and treatment mean that they are ideally placed to address the physical, behavioural, occupational, psychosocial and emotional impact of pain. This requires therapists to draw on their full repertoire of skills, broadening their focus beyond the mere elimination of the person's pain and instead helping someone to live better *despite* pain.

Resources

Arthritis Care (2011) *Arthritis Hurts: The Emotional Impact of Pain*. Online Survey.

Arthritis Research UK (2010) *Sexuality and Arthritis*. www.arthritiscare.org.uk/@2118/copy_of_ArthritisHurts. Accessed on 19 November 2012.

British Pain Society is involved in all aspects of pain and its management. http://www.britishpainsociety.org/book_understanding_pain.pdf. Accessed on 14 November 2012.

Change Pain is a non-promotional web-based education programme from Grünenthal, a research-based pharmaceutical company that specialises in the management of pain. http://www.change-pain.co.uk/cme/specialist-modules/cbt/. Accessed on 14 November 2012.

Cochrane review on *Psychological Therapy for Adults with Longstanding Distressing Pain and Disability*. http://summaries.cochrane.org/CD007407/psychological-therapy-for-adults-with-longstanding-distressing-pain-and-disability. Accessed on 14 November 2012.

David L (2010) Cognitive behavioural approaches to chronic pain in primary care, Change Pain, Education Modules (CME) Series.

Getting to GRIPS with Chronic Pain in Scotland – a report that is benchmarking Chronic Pain Services in Partnership with NHS Boards, Patients and Service Providers. http://www. nospg.nhsscotland.com/wp-content/05_12-RDP-report-on-Chronic-Pain.pdf. Accessed on 14 November 2012.

International Association for the Study of Pain (IASP) is a professional forum for science, practice and education in the field of pain. http://www.iasp-pain.org//AM/Template. cfm?Section=Home. Accessed on 14 November 2012.

Moorthy A (2011) Rheumatoid arthritis, Change Pain, case study Education Module (CME) Series. http://www.change-pain.co.uk/cme/case-studies/rheumatoid-arthritis/. Accessed on 14 November 2012.

Live Well – Psychological techniques for coping with pain. http://www.nhs.uk/Livewell/Pain/ Pages/10painself-helptips.aspx. Accessed on 14 November 2012.

National Pain Audit. http://nationalpainaudit.org/media/files/GRIPS_booklet.pdf. Accessed on 14 November 2012.

NHS Quality Improvement Scotland (2nd edn.) July 2008.

Pain Toolkit – A website for people who live with persistent pain. http://www.paintoolkit.org/. Accessed on 14 November 2012.

Relaxation – Relaxation techniques are described in various books, but Payne R (2000) *Relaxation Techniques: A Practical Handbook for the Health Care Professional* (2nd edn.). London: Churchill Livingstone and Strong J (1996) *Chronic Pain: The Occupational Therapists Perspective*. London: Churchill Livingstone are particularly useful resources for therapists.

Sex and Arthritis. http://www.arthritisresearchuk.org/~/media/Files/Arthritis-information/ Living-with-arthritis/2037-Sex-and-arthritis.ashx. Accessed on 14 November 2012.

References

Affleck G, Tennen H, Pfeiffer C, et al. (1987) Appraisals of control and predictability in adapting to a chronic disease. *Journal of Personality and Social Psychology* 53(2):273–279.

Affleck G, Tennen H, Urrows S, et al. (1994) Person and contextual features of daily stress reactivity: Individual differences in relations of undesirable daily events with mood disturbance in chronic pain intensity. *Journal of Personality and Social Psychology* 94:329–360.

Alsaker S, Bongaardt R, Josephsson S (2009) Studying narrative-in-action in women with chronic rheumatic conditions. *Qualitative Health Research* 19:1154–1161.

Ashburn M, Staats P (1999) Management of chronic pain. *Lancet* 5353:1865–1869.

Astin JA, Bedkner M, Wright K (2002) Psychological interventions in rheumatoid arthritis: A meta-analysis of randomised controlled trials. *Arthritis Care and Research* 47(3):291–302.

Backman CL (2006) Arthritis and pain. Psychological aspects in the management of arthritis pain. *Arthritis Research Therapy* 8:221.

Baer R (2005) *Mindfulness-Based Treatment Approaches: Clinician's Guide to Evidence Base and Applications* (1st edn.). New York: Academic Press.

Barlow J (2009) *Living with Arthritis*. Oxford, UK: The British Psychological Society, BPS Blackwell.

Beck JS (2006) Cognitive-behavioural therapy (interview). *Primary Psychiatry* 13(4):31–34.

Birkholtz M, Aylwin L, Harman R (2004) Activity pacing in chronic pain management: One aim, but which methods? Part One: Introduction and literature review. *British Journal of Occupational Therapy* 67(10):447–452.

Bliddal H (2007) Chronic widespread pain in the spectrum of rheumatological diseases. *Best Practice Research Clinical Rheumatology* 21:91–402.

Bury M (1991) The Sociology of chronic illness: A review of research and prospects. *Sociology of Health & Illness* 13(4):451–468.

Butler D, Moseley GL (2003) *Explain Pain*. Adelaide, Australia: NOI Group Publishing.

Carroll D, Seers K (1998) Relaxation for the relief of chronic pain: A systematic review. *Journal of Advanced Nursing* 27:476–487.

Cole F, Macdonald H, Carus, et al. (2005) *Overcoming Chronic Pain – A Self Help Guide to Using Cognitive Behavioural Techniques*. London: Robinson.

Creed F, Ash G (1992) Depression in rheumatoid arthritis: Aetiology and treatment. *International Review of Psychiatry* 4:23–34.

David L (2006) *Using CBT in General Practice: The 10 Minute Consultation*. Bloxham, UK: Scion Publishing Ltd.

David L (2010) *Cognitive Behavioural Approaches to Chronic Pain in Primary Care, Change Pain, Education Modules (CME) Series*. http://www.change-pain.co.uk/cme/specialist-modules/cbt/. Accessed on 11 November 2012.

Dickens C, McGowan L, Clark-Carter D, et al. (2002) Depression in rheumatoid arthritis: A systematic review of the literature with meta-analysis. *Psychosomatic Medicine* 64(1):52–60.

Dubouloz CJ, Laporte D, Hall M, et al. (2004) Transformation of meaning perspectives in clients with rheumatoid arthritis. *American Journal of Occupational Therapy* 58:398–407.

Dubouloz CJ, Vallerand J, Laporte D, et al. (2008) Occupational performance modification and personal change among clients receiving rehabilitation services for rheumatoid arthritis. *Australian Occupational Therapy Journal* 55:30–38.

Elenkov IJ (2008) Neurohormonal-cytokine interactions: Implications for inflammation, common human diseases and well-being. *Neurochemistry International* 52:40–51.

Evers AWM, Kraaimaat FW, van Riel RPLCM, et al. (2002) Tailored cognitive behavioural therapy in early RA for patients at risk: An RCT. *Pain* 100:141–153.

Furst GP, Gerber LH, Smith CC, et al. (1987) A program for improving energy conservation behaviors in adults with rheumatoid arthritis. *American Journal of Occupational Therapy* 41:102–111.

Gatchel R, Peng Y, Peters M, et al. (2007) The biopsychosocial approach to chronic pain: Scientific advances and future directions. *Psychological Bulletin* 133(4):581–624.

Gilworth G, Woodhouse A, Tennant A, et al. (2001) The impact of rheumatoid arthritis in the workplace. *British Journal of Therapy and Rehabilitation* 8(9):342–347.

Germer CK (2005) Mindfulness: What is it? What does it matter? In: Germer CK, Siegel RD, Fulton PR (eds.) *Mindfulness and Psychotherapy* (pp. 3–27). New York: Guildford Press.

Greenberger D, Padesky CA (1995) *Mind Over Mood*. New York/London: The Guildford Press.

Grossman P, Tiefenthaler-Gilmer U, Raysz A, et al. (2007) Mindfulness training as an interventions for fibromyalgia: Evidence of post-intervention and 3 year follow up benefits in well-being. *Psychotherapy and Psychosomatics* 76(4):226–233.

Hammond A, Reeve LJ, McArthur MA (2008) Occupational therapy in musculoskeletal chronic pain management. In: *British Society for Rheumatology and IASP Musculoskeletal Pain Taskforce guidelines for the Integrated Management of Musculoskeletal Pain Symptoms*

(IMMsPS) (pp. 158–66). http://www.hope-academic.org.uk/Academic/researchdevelopment/Themes/Neurosciences/Pain/Guidelines_for_the_Management_of_Musculoskeletal_Pain_FINA.pdf. Accessed on 11 November 2012.

Hawtin H, Sullivan C (2011) Experiences of mindfulness training in living with rheumatic disease: An interpretative phenomenological analysis. *British Journal of Occupational Therapy* 74(3):137–142.

Hewlett S, Chalder T, Choy E, et al. (2011) Fatigue in rheumatoid arthritis: Time for a conceptual model. *Rheumatology* 50:1004–1006.

Hughes J (2009) Exploring the impact of rheumatoid arthritis on patients' lives. *International Journal of Therapy and Rehabilitation* 16(11):594–599.

International Association for the Study of Pain (IASP) (2011) *Terminology Review*.. http://www.iasp-pain.org/AM/Template.cfm?Section=General_Resource_Links&Template=/CM/HTMLDisplay.cfm&ContentID=3058. Accessed on 23 November 2012.

Katz WA, Rottenberg (2005) The nature of pain: Pathophysiology. *Journal of Clinical Rheumatology* 11(52):11–15.

Katz PP, Yelin EH (1993) Prevalence and correlates of depressive symptoms among persons with rheumatoid arthritis. *Journal of Rheumatology* 20(5):790–796.

Keable D (1997) *The Management of Anxiety: A Guide for Therapists* (2nd edn.). New York: Churchill Livingstone.

Kett C, Flint J, Openshaw M, et al. (2010) Self-management strategies used during flares of rheumatoid arthritis in an ethnically diverse population. *Musculoskeletal Care* 8(4):204–214.

Kojima M, Suzuki S, Furukawa TA, et al. (2009) Depression, inflammation and pain in patients with rheumatoid arthritis. *Arthritis and Rheumatism* 61(8):1018–1024.

Lamberg L (1999) Chronic pain linked with poor sleep; exploration of causes and treatment. *Journal of the American Medical Association* 281:691–692.

Locker D (1983) *Disability and Disadvantage: The Consequences of Chronic Illness*. London/New York: Tavistock Publications.

Macedo AM, Oakley SP, Panayi GS, et al. (2009) Functional and work outcomes improve in patients with rheumatoid arthritis who receive targeted, comprehensive occupational therapy. *Arthritis and Rheumatism (Arthritis Care and Research)* 61(11):1522–1530.

MacKichan F, Wylde V, Dieppe P (2008) The assessment of musculoskeletal pain in the clinical setting. *Rheumatic Diseases Clinical North America* 34:311–330.

Main CJ, Williams AC (2002) Musculoskeletal pain. *British Medical Journal* 325:534–537.

Mann EM, Carr ECJ (2009) *Pain: Creative Approaches to Effective Management* (2nd edn.). London: Palgrave Macmillan.

McCracken LM, Vowles KE (2006) Acceptance of chronic pain. *Current Pain and Headache Reports* 10(2):90–94.

McKenna J (2007) Emotional intelligence training in adjustment to physical disability and illness. *International Journal of Therapy and Rehabilitation* 14(12):551–556.

Melvin J, Jensen G (eds.) (2000) *Rheumatologic Rehabilitation Series: Vol. 1. Assessment and Management*. Bethesda, MD: American Occupational Therapy Association.

Mengshoel AM (2008) Living with a fluctuating illness of ankylosing spondylitis: A qualitative study. *Arthritis and Rheumatism (Arthritis Care and Research)* 59(10):1439–1444.

Milne JM (1983) The biopsychosocial model as applied to a multidisciplinary pain management programme. *Journal of New Zealand Association of Occupational Therapists* 34:19–21.

Minnock P, Bresnihan B (2004) Pain outcome and fatigue levels reported by women with established rheumatoid arthritis. *Arthritis Rheumatism* 50(Suppl 9):S471.5.

Montecucco C, Cavagna L, Campbell R (2009) Pain and rheumatology: An overview of the problem. *European Journal of Pain Supplements* 3:105–109.

National Institute of Clinical Excellence (NICE) (2009) *Rheumatoid Arthritis: National Clinical Guideline for Management and Treatment in Adults.* London: Royal College of Physicians.

National Rheumatoid Arthritis Society (NRAS) (2004) *Beyond the Pain: The Social and Psychological Impact of RA.* http://www.nras.org.uk/. Accessed on 11 November 2012.

NRAS (2007) *I Want to Work: Employment and Rheumatoid Arthritis: A National Picture.* NRAS Survey. http://www.nras.org.uk/help_for_you/publications/publication_detail.aspx?id=a0B80000005CJTdEAO. Accessed on 11 November 12.

NRAS (2010) *RA and Work: Scottish Work Survey.* NRAS Survey. http://www.nras.org.uk/help_for_you/publications/publication_detail.aspx?id=a0B8000000A9aaCEAR. Accessed on 11 November 2012.

Newman S, Fitzpatrick R, Revenson TA, et al. (1996) *Understanding Rheumatoid Arthritis.* London/New York: Routledge.

O'Hara P (1996) *Pain Management for Health Professionals.* London: Chapman & Hall.

Parsons G, Preece W (2010) *Principles and Practice of Managing Pain: A Guide for Nurses and Allied Health Professionals.* Berkshire, UK: McGraw Hill, Open University Press.

Payne R (2000) *Relaxation Techniques: A Practical Handbook for the Health Care Professional* (2nd edn.), New York: Churchill Livingstone.

Penny KI, Purves AM, Smith BH, et al. (1999) Relationship between chronic pain grade and measures of physical, social and psychological well-being. *Pain* 79:275–279.

Persson D, Andersson I, Eklund M (2011) Defying Aches and reevaluating daily doing: Occupational perspectives on adjusting to chronic pain. *Scandinavian Journal of Occupational Therapy* 18:188–197.

Pradhan EK, Baumgarten M, Langenberg P, et al. (2007) Effect of mindfulness based stress reduction in rheumatoid arthritis patients. *Arthritis and Rheumatism (Arthritis Care and Research)* 57(7):1134–1142.

Reisine ST, Goodenow C, Grady KE (1987) The impact of Rheumatoid arthritis on the home-maker. *Social Science and Medicine* 25(1):89–95.

Riemsma RP, Rasker JJ, Taal E, et al. (1998) Fatigue in rheumatoid arthritis: The role of self-efficacy and problematic social support. *British Journal of Rheumatology* 37:1042–1046.

Rogers CR (1959) A theory of therapy, personality, and interpersonal relationships as develop in the client-centred framework. In: Koch S (ed.) *Psychology: The Study of Science: Vol. 3. Formulations of the Person and the Social Contexts.* New York: McGraw-Hill.

Rosenbaum RB (2001) Neuromuscular complications of connective tissue diseases. *Muscle Nerve* 24:154–169.

Sandles L (1990) *Occupational Therapy in Rheumatology – An Holistic Approach.* London: Chapman and Hall.

Seers C, Friedli K (1996) The patients' experience of their chonic non-malignant pain. *Journal of Advanced Nursing* 24:1160–1168.

Sheane BJ, Doyle F, Doyle C, et al. (2008) Sub-optimal pain control in patients with rheumatic disease. *Clinical Rheumatology* 27:829–839.

Shlotzhauer TL, McGuire JL (2003) *Living with Rheumatoid Arthritis* (2nd edn.). Baltimore, MD/London: The John Hopkins University Press.

Skevington SM (1998) Investigating the relationship between pain and discomfort and quality of life using the WHOQOL. *Pain* 76:395–406.

Skjutar A, Schult M, Christensson K, et al. (2010) Indicators of need for occupational therapy inpatients with chronic pain: Occupational therapists' focus groups. *Occupational Therapy International* 17:93–103.

Stamm TA, Wright J, Machold K, et al. (2004) Occupational balance of women with rheumatoid arthritis: A qualitative study. *Musculoskeletal Care* 2(2):101–112.

Steutjens EEMJ, Dejjer JJ, Bouter LM, et al. (2008) *Occupational Therapy for Rheumatoid Arthritis (Review)*. Chichester, UK: The Cochrane Collaboration, John Wiley & Sons Ltd. www.thecochranelibrary.com. Accessed on 11 November 2012.

Stout K, Finlayson M (2011) Fatigue management in chronic illness: The role of the occupational therapist. *American Occupational Therapy* 24(1):16–19. www.aota.org. Accessed on 11 November 2012.

Strong J (1996) *Chronic Pain: The Occupational Therapists Perspective*. London: Churchill Livingstone.

Strong J (2002) Lifestyle management. In: Strong J, Unruh AM, Wright A, Baxter GD (eds.) *Pain: A Textbook for Therapists*. London: Churchill Livingstone.

Strong J, Unruh AM, Wright A, et al. (eds.) (2002) *Pain: A Textbook for Therapists*. London: Churchill Livingstone.

Summers MN, Haley WE, Reveille JD, et al. (1988) Radiographic assessment and psychologic variables as predictors of pain and functional impairment in osteoarthritis of the knee or hip. *Arthritis and Rheumatism* 31(2):204–209.

Taylor-Gjevre RM, Gjevre JA, Nair B, et al. (2011) Components of sleep quality and sleep fragmentation in rheumatoid arthritis and osteoarthritis. *Musculoskeletal Care* 9(3):152–159.

Thompson B (2009) Mindfulness-based stress reduction for people with chronic conditions. *British Journal of Occupational Therapy* 72(9):405–410.

Vroman K, Warner R, Chamberlain K (2009) Now let me tell you in my own words: Narratives of acute and chronic low back pain. *Disability and Rehabilitation* 31(12):967–987.

Wall P (1999) *Pain – The Science of Suffering*. London: Phoenix.

Wells C, Nown G (1993) *The Pain Relief Handbook – Self Help Methods for Managing Pain*. London: Vermilion.

World Health Organisation (WHO) (2003) The burden of musculoskeletal conditions at the start of the millennium. *World Health Organisation Technical Report Series* 919:1–218.

Wiener CL (1975) The burden of tolerating uncertainty. *Social Science and Medicine* 9:97–104.

Wolfe F, Michaud K (2009) Predicting depression in rheumatoid arthritis: The signal importance of pain extent and fatigue, and co-morbidity. *Arthritis and Rheumatism* 61:667–673.

Wright A, Benson H, O'Callaghan (2002) Pharmacology of pain management. In: Strong J, Unruh AM, Wright A, Baxter GD (eds.) *Pain: A Textbook for Therapists*. New York: Churchill Livingstone.

Yeung R (2010) *The Extra One Per Cent: How Small Changes Make Exceptional People*. London: Pan Macmillan.

Zautra ZJ, Davis MC, Reich JW, et al. (2008) Comparison of cognitive behavioural and mindfulness meditation interventions on adaptation to rheumatoid arthritis for patient with and without history of depression. *Journal of Consulting and Clinical Psychology* 77(3):408–421.

Chapter 10

Maintaining independence

Jill Jepson[1] and Lynne Goodacre[2]

[1]University of East Anglia, Norfolk, United Kingdom; [2]Lancaster University, Lancaster, United Kingdom

10.1 Introduction

Assistive technology (AT) and environmental adaptation have the potential to increase independence, reduce the need for personal assistance and prevent or reduce health problems (Office of the Deputy Prime Minister 2005). Due to the levels of activity limitation experienced by people with rheumatic conditions, assessment for and recommendation of AT is a key focus of occupational therapy practice in rheumatology (COT 2003; Hammond 2004). The rationale for AT use by people with rheumatic conditions comprises increasing or maintaining independence, reducing pain and fatigue associated with undertaking a task, minimising biomechanical stress and forces placed on joints during activity, minimising the risks associated with undertaking a task and providing assistance to carers.

Whilst assessment for AT and environmental adaptation is a central component of practice, three factors are currently influencing this area of practice: the increasing use of biologic therapies in the treatment of inflammatory arthritis which may reduce the amount of AT required; the increasing adoption of an inclusive approach to the design of mainstream products; and the shifting trend towards the retail model of AT supply. Whilst the first two may lead to a reduction in the need for AT, the latter has significant implications for how AT is acquired by people with rheumatic conditions.

In this chapter, we will explore the reasons for non-use of AT and introduce the Matching Person and Technology (MPT) model as a framework for assessment which has the potential to minimise non-use. We will illustrate how this model can be applied to the assessment of people with rheumatic conditions and explore different models of AT service provision. We will then explore how AT, home adaptation

Rheumatology Practice in Occupational Therapy: Promoting Lifestyle Management, First Edition.
Edited by Lynne Goodacre and Margaret McArthur.
© 2013 John Wiley & Sons, Ltd. Published 2013 by John Wiley & Sons, Ltd.

and inclusive design can be utilised to overcome activity limitation and maximise independence in people with rheumatic conditions.

10.2   What is assistive technology?

The term 'assistive technology' has replaced the expression disability equipment to describe products and services used by people of all ages to gain increased autonomy and maximise their occupational performance (FAST 2012). Alternative definitions focus on defining the outcomes required by users of AT and have identified that assistive devices and services should improve the ease and safety with which occupations are carried out (Cowan and Turner Smith 1999; WHO 2004). The use of AT can be linked to the domains of the International Classification of Functioning, Disability and Health (ICF) (WHO 2001) in order to clarify the outcomes that an individual may wish to achieve. AT can be used to compensate for or relieve impairment of body function or structure, e.g. the use of an orthosis to relieve pain in a joint; to reduce activity limitations, e.g. use of a walking stick to aid mobility; enable participation in daily occupations, e.g. car adaptations to enable an individual to drive to work; and reduce the barriers presented by an environment, e.g. automatic doors to facilitate access to public buildings (Bougie 2003; Karlsson 2003).

AT is not an end in itself but one tool that can enable people with occupational dysfunction to achieve their personal goals. AT may offer an individual the tools for autonomy through independence in daily life, self-determination, participation and identification (Van de Ven et al. 2008), but it can only be successfully used if underpinned by accurate and comprehensive assessment and the required level of ongoing support.

10.3   Reducing non-use of assistive technology

The evidence base for the effectiveness of AT remains limited with the majority of studies investigating non-use or abandonment of devices rather than efficacy (de Boer et al. 2009; Hocking 1999; Ripat and Booth 2005; Wessels et al. 2003). A Cochrane review of AT for rheumatoid arthritis (Tuntland et al. 2009) highlighted the paucity of evidence for the use of AT by people with rheumatic conditions.

Studies of non-use of AT suggest that up to a third of all products provided are not used (Scherer 2002). The factors identified as affecting non-use have been categorised into personal, device related, environmental and intervention related (Wessels et al. 2003). Personal factors include characteristics such as age, gender and disability, expectations of occupational performance, self-image and changes in functional abilities. Device-related factors include the quality and performance of the device as well as the aesthetics and design features. Environmental factors encompass societal and economic issues as well as service provision and choice; intervention factors include

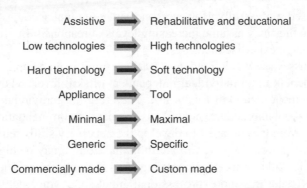

Assistive ➡	Rehabilitative and educational
Low technologies ➡	High technologies
Hard technology ➡	Soft technology
Appliance ➡	Tool
Minimal ➡	Maximal
Generic ➡	Specific
Commercially made ➡	Custom made

Figure 10.1   Characterisation of ATs. (Adapted from Cook and Hussey 2002.)

the user's involvement in decision making, assessment and support for AT (Ripat and Booth 2005; Wessels et al. 2003).

This list of reasons for non-use highlights the importance of skilled assessment and user involvement alongside a clear understanding of the important features and desired outcomes of AT devices. In order to properly assess for and recommend AT, as well as to support individuals in using AT devices, it is helpful to develop a structured way of thinking about and defining ATs. The diversity of devices and services is far reaching, and a classification framework devised by Cook and Hussey (2002) is helpful when considering all aspects of assessment and provision.

Classification of AT

Cook and Hussey (2002) suggest that all ATs can be classified from a set of perspectives that represent a spectrum on which AT can be judged (Figure 10.1). The use of this classification framework can assist in identifying some key considerations that inform the assessment for and provision of AT and highlight some potential reasons for non-use or abandonment.

Some of the classifications are relatively self-explanatory; AT devices can be used to augment or replace function (assistive) or be used as a therapeutic tool (rehabilitative). A low-technology device is relatively simple, inexpensive and easy to maintain in comparison to a high-technology device. A generic AT device can be used for a number of functions whilst a specific device is function specific, e.g. a night resting splint; AT devices can be purchased off the shelf or designed and developed for a specific individual, in which case aftercare and support become critical considerations. However, other classifications need more careful consideration.

The classification of hard and soft technologies may help with identifying the support required to prevent non-use; hard technologies representing the device or system; and soft technologies the human input for decision making, support and training. The therapist will initially take the lead with soft technology input, using their knowledge and skills as a professional to ensure that the hard technology can be obtained and used successfully. However, once an individual becomes an experienced user of a device they may assume increasing levels of responsibility for the soft technology side as their expertlse increases.

Cook and Hussey use Vanderheiden's (1991) definition of an appliance as 'a device that provides benefit to an individual independent of skill level' whereas a tool may require development of a skill for its use. Therefore, an individual who is recommended to use a tool may require not only assessment, recommendation and fitting of AT but support from the therapist to develop the necessary skills required to use the AT device, e.g. a powered scooter. In addition, the 'tools' may be highly specialised and therefore the skills for usage cannot be gained from observing other people using the tools, thus requiring more professional input, e.g. voice-activated computer software.

The classification of AT on a spectrum from minimal to maximal prompts consideration of the level of need as a function of the AT that will guide the assessment, recommendation and support process. Minimal technology tends to augment rather than replace function with maximal need representing high levels of dependency on an AT device. If need is identified as on the maximal end of the spectrum, then the quality and performance of the device and the accuracy of assessment for purpose will be critical to successful and continued usage.

10.4   Matching person and technology

The MPT model and associated assessment tools (Scherer 2000) provide a structured approach to improving the fit between the needs of an individual requiring an AT intervention and the recommended device in order to ensure improved outcomes and reduced abandonment of AT. The process focuses on three main areas for consideration and assessment when recommending an AT intervention which reflect the identified reasons for non-use or abandonment of AT. The MPT process requires the therapist to consider the client's personal and psychosocial needs and preferences, the environment or milieu in which AT will be used and the essential and desirable features and functions of the required AT (Scherer et al. 2005). Examples of issues for assessment and consideration can be seen in Figure 10.2.

The MPT model represents a collaborative process between the service user and the therapist. The aim is to identify and assess the factors and features that will contribute to the recommendation of the most appropriate product for an individual, thus reducing the likelihood of inappropriate provision, client dissatisfaction and consequent non-use.

The Institute for Matching Person and Technology (http://www.matchingperson-andtechnology.com/index.html) have identified a six-step approach to AT assessment and produced a series of assessment instruments that can be modified for use in the UK. The instruments include the Survey of Technology Use to identify technologies which a person feels comfortable using to enable new technology to match level of comfort or success. There are also four technology-specific instruments focusing on

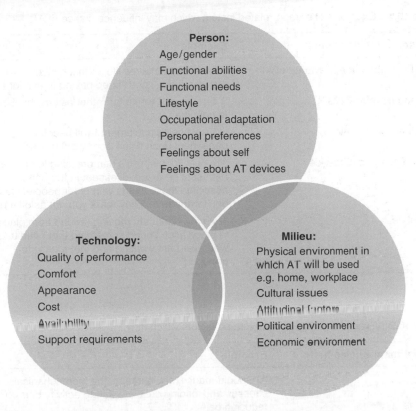

Person:
Age/gender
Functional abilities
Functional needs
Lifestyle
Occupational adaptation
Personal preferences
Feelings about self
Feelings about AT devices

Technology:
Quality of performance
Comfort
Appearance
Cost
Availability
Support requirements

Milieu:
Physical environment in
which AT will be used
e.g. home, workplace
Cultural issues
Attitudinal factors
Political environment
Economic environment

Figure 10.2 Issues for assessment and consideration

AT, workplace technology, educational technology and healthcare technology. Each instrument comprises two tools, one for the user and one for the therapist.

10.5 Applying the MPT to AT for people with rheumatic conditions

In this section the MPT framework is used to illustrate factors relevant to the assessment of people with rheumatic conditions. Before undertaking an assessment for AT, consideration should be given as to whether this is the most effective intervention. The identified activity limitation may be overcome by utilising principles of joint protection and/or pacing, e.g. the reorganisation of the environment, the delegation of a task to another person and/or the completion of an activity in several stages.

Person-related factors

A crucial factor to establish early in the assessment process is a person's predisposition to AT use. Using AT often requires behaviour change and the Trans-Theoretical

Table 10.1   Examples of person-related factors which may influence choice of AT.

Person-related factors	Example
Feelings about the relevance of AT	'These things makes life so much easier, they are wonderful. I don't keep having to ask for help'
Personal preferences	'If I get stuck I would far rather ask my husband to help me'
Feelings about self	'If I start using equipment I will become dependent upon it so I don't want to start'
Feelings about AT devices	'I'm only 30. I think it's demoralising to have a bath seat or raised toilet seat in the house. You associate those things with older people. I just don't want them. They mark you out as different'
Lifestyle	'With my work I am moving around from place to place a lot. I need something that I can use wherever I am working and that it easy to transport'

Table 10.2   Examples of impairment-related factors which may influence choice of AT.

Impairment-related factors	Example
Pain	AT should reduce, not increase, the biomechanical stresses and loading on joints during activity thus reducing pain
Stiffness	The presence of morning stiffness can have a significant impact on performance; this must be borne in mind during assessment and/or indicate the best time to assess
Fatigue	AT may be recommended to reduce the effort expended in tasks such as dressing, bathing, meal preparation
Variability	Consideration should be given to how an exacerbation or progression of the impairment may affect AT use, i.e. can a change in ability be accommodated or will an alternative be required. Regular and ongoing assessment may also be indicated during times of high variability
Loss or limitation in movement	Limited movement and reduced strength in upper or lower limbs can increase the difficulty of using the AT, e.g. transferring onto a bed if hip and knee movement is restricted
Reduced hand function	Attention should be paid to the kind of device controls and grips to identify whether alternatives are needed to accommodate poor hand function
Subcutaneous nodules	AT should not place pressure on the nodules if they exist.
Skin integrity	Long-term use of steroids can affect skin integrity and shear on the skin needs to be considered with certain products especially where the skin is in direct contact with the product, i.e. bathing equipment

Table 10.3 Examples of product-related factors which may influence choice of AT.

Product-related factors	Example
Weight of product	Especially important if the product needs to be moved on a regular basis
Weight of person	Is the person within the weight limits of the product?
Portability	If the item needs to be transported, the ease with which this can be done must be considered along with implications for additional AT to facilitate transportation, i.e. hoist to lift powered scooter into boot of car
Storage	If items need to be stored, their ability to fold or dismantle should be considered alongside appropriate storage facilities.
Comfort	Weight loss or nodules can cause discomfort, especially when sitting on hard surfaces for any length of time, thought should be given to the need for padding and pressure relief
Usability	Is fitting/ demonstration and/or training required and if so who is going to do this? Are the controls easy to use? Does the AT require regular charging and servicing? Does the AT support the principles of joint protection?
Aesthetics	Is the appearance and design of the product acceptable to the client?
Cost	If being purchased privately is the cost of the product within the resources of the client or is a cheaper alternative or additional funding required? If the device requires a special purchase through statutory authorities, the use of sound clinical reasoning will be required to justify the extra cost

Model (see Chapter 7) can be applied to the introduction and use of AT to determine when and how it is introduced and the level and type of support required. If a person is resistant to AT, it is likely to be abandoned unless they develop an understanding of its relevance. If a person is amenable to AT use but the AT is perceived to be complex without training and support, it may not be used in the long term. Therefore, careful consideration needs to be given to addressing the influence of person-related factors as illustrated by the examples of people talking about using AT (Table 10.1).

A range of person-specific impairment-related factors also need to be considered which focus on the aspects of rheumatic conditions which may influence product selection (Table 10.2)

Product-related factors

Due to the increasing range of AT it is likely that once a specific need for AT is identified there will be a range of products from which to choose. A number of factors should be taken into consideration (Table 10.3).

Table 10.4   Examples of environment-related factors which may influence choice of AT.

Environment-related factors	Example
Physical environment in which AT will be used	Can the environment accommodate the AT, e.g. can the material the bath is made of support a bath seat, can the walls accommodate fixed rails?
Cultural issues	What are the cultural values of the environment, e.g. is the workplace culture enabling and supportive? Are there cultural issues with regard to tasks for which AT may be used, e.g. hygiene
Attitudinal factors	Who else is using the environment? How do they respond to the AT? Does the AT inhibit other people using the environment, e.g. the bath or the toilet?
Political environment	Does the current political climate support provision of AT for a particular purpose, e.g. return to work, reduction of care costs?
Economic environment	Is the required AT able to be funded from statutory funding?
	How can the use of AT improve the economic prospects of the service user?

Environment-related factors

The majority of AT will be used either within a person's home or their place of work; therefore, it needs to be compatible with whichever environment it is going to be used in (Table 10.4).

10.6   Assistive technology outcomes

Outcome measures are important from the perspectives of both the service user and the service provider to ensure satisfaction with the AT recommended, and to achieve continuous improvement of the services for people requiring AT interventions. The two most commonly used AT-specific outcome measures are the Quebec User Evaluation of Satisfaction with Assistive Technology (QUEST 2.0) and the Psychosocial Impact of Assistive Devices Scale (PIADS).

Quebec User Evaluation of Satisfaction with Assistive Technology (QUEST 2.0)

QUEST 2.0 is based on the MPT model designed to evaluate user reported satisfaction with an AT device using a multidimensional measure (Demers et al. 2002a), comprising satisfaction with the Device and the Services. The Device dimension requires users to evaluate satisfaction with comfort, weight, durability, adjustments, simplicity of use, dimensions, effectiveness and safety. The Service dimension requires users to evaluate satisfaction with delivery, professional service, follow-up and repairs and servicing.

Each item is rated on a five-point scale with a final question requiring the user to identify the 3 most important items from the 12 listed. The scale can be administered in self-complete format or by an interviewer using optional interactive materials and has also been evaluated as a postal survey (Goodacre and Turner 2005). The evaluation questionnaire takes 10–15 min per device to complete (Demers et al. 2002b).

Psychosocial Impact of Assistive Devices Scale (PIADS)

PIADS© (Day and Jutai 1996) is designed to be a generic evaluation of any form of AT device and evaluates user satisfaction with AT across three dimensions: adaptability (the enabling effect of the device in relation to the willingness to try new things); competence (feelings of usefulness, performance and productivity) and self-esteem (emotional well-being and happiness). PIADS can be used with people of all ages and abilities and has been translated into 14 languages.

In addition to these two measures that focus on user satisfaction with an AT device, a more recent outcome measure has been developed in the Netherlands to assess the quality of service delivery which, as shown earlier in this chapter, is integral to successful AT provision. KWAZO (Dijcks et al. 2006) is a questionnaire that requires the AT user to grade the provider as insufficient, sufficient and good on seven criteria:

- Accessibility
- Information
- Co-ordination
- Know-how
- Efficiency
- Participation
- Instruction

The service provider service receives a score between 7 and 21, with a high score reflecting a high level of satisfaction with the service and a score of 14 a generally sufficient service. The questionnaire has been translated into English but is currently only validated in Dutch and Finnish (Ahtola et al. 2011).

Finally, the more generic Canadian Occupational Performance Measure (COPM 4th Ed) is commonly used as an outcome measure of satisfaction with AT across a range of different devices (Giesbrecht et al. 2009; Petty et al. 2005; Ripat 2006; Wessels et al. 2004). COPM is used to detect change in a client's self-perception of occupational performance before and after provision of AT. It can be used with people with many different disabilities and is frequently used in conjunction with an AT-specific outcome measure.

10.7   Methods of obtaining AT

It is not the intention of this section to engage with the mechanisms for funding and service provision with regard to AT and home adaptations as this is beyond the scope of this chapter; relevant links to such information are provided for those who require them. Information is provided however on recent changes impacting on the ability of people with rheumatic conditions to access such services.

The retail model

In 2006, a further review of community equipment services led to the formation of the Department of Health Transforming Community Equipment Services Team who recommended the introduction of a retail model of community equipment for 'simple aids to daily living'. Within this model, a person's statutory right to assessment is retained but therapists identifying an AT need are required to write a prescription which can be exchanged with an approved retailer who is responsible for supply and, where appropriate, fitting.

A 3-year project currently being undertaken by ASSIST UK and Ricability is utilising 'mystery shoppers' to determine the quality of service provided by retailers of AT. Whilst finding the quality of service to be generally good, with some exceptions, the project has highlighted that obtaining sufficient information to make informed choices about the right product is often reliant upon the customer asking sufficiently informed questions as retailers had a tendency to overestimate the customer's knowledge (Assist UK and Ricability 2011). Therefore, whether a client is obtaining AT from a retailer via a prescription or private purchase they need expert guidance to inform their selection.

The Self-Assessment Rapid Access Project (SARA)

Many of the difficulties experienced by people with rheumatic conditions, whilst having the potential to impact negatively on their quality of life, are not, in service provider terms, perceived as high priority. Increasingly, people are experiencing difficulty obtaining funding for AT and home adaptations, as well as lengthy delays for assessment and supply or completion of work. Increasingly, therefore, clients are choosing to fund their own AT and home adaptation work. For people choosing this option, it is essential to ensure that they are equipped with relevant information about sources of advice and guidance to ensure that they obtain the most appropriate solution to the problem they are experiencing.

SARA developed by the Disabled Living Foundation (DLF) is designed to enable users to conduct their own self-assessment online. The system via a series of questions relevant to the problem they have identified leads people through a self-assessment process and then provides a comprehensive list of suggestions for possible solutions with links to relevant services in the statutory and independent sectors. The SARA system has also been customised for and is being used by some local authorities.

Trusted Assessor Framework

Within the reviews of community equipment services, emphasis was placed on improved training for service providers to enable a wider range of people to be able to assess for and provide AT. In 2005, the Trusted Assessor Framework (Winchcombe and Ballinger 2005) project established the competencies required to enable support workers to assess for less complex items of AT, many of which are relevant to people with rheumatic conditions.

10.8 Commonly used AT and home adaptations for people with rheumatic conditions

Covering the range of AT and home adaptations applicable to people with rheumatic conditions is beyond the scope of a single chapter, and therefore examples have been provided of how some areas of activity limitation experienced by people with rheumatic conditions may be addressed either within mainstream design, via the use of AT or via home adaptation (Tables 10.5, 10.6 and 10.7).

10.9 Inclusive design

'Inclusive design' is the term used to describe a design process whereby designers 'address the needs of the widest possible audience by including the needs of groups who are currently excluded from or marginalised by mainstream design practices' (Design Council Living Longer 2012). In the early 1990s, it was recognised that much design innovation was focused on the needs of younger people, and the dangers of excluding many groups of people from the design process were being challenged (Coleman 2006). Design exclusion impacts on all aspects of peoples' lives and occurs in homes, workplaces, transportations systems, retail environments, public spaces and leisure facilities.

One of the key drivers for inclusive design has been the realisation of the economic implications of continuing to exclude a significant and growing proportion of the population from the design process. The expanding ageing population represents a significant sector of society with disposable income, and companies integrating the

Table 10.5 Personal care and hygiene.

Activity limitation	Mainstream design	Assistive technology	Home adaptation
Bathing	Modern wet room area	Portable bath lift	Level access shower with shower seat
Toileting	Wall-mounted toilet installed at the appropriate height	Raised toilet seat	Toilet plinth fitted between floor and toilet to raise height
Personal hygiene	Bidet	Bottom wiper	Electric bidet with wash/dry facility
Personal care	Powered toothbrush/shaver	Tubing to enlarge grip, easy grip handles	

Table 10.6   Food preparation and household tasks.

Activity limitation	Mainstream design	Assistive technology	Housing adaptation
Standing tolerance	Energy-saving kitchen layout	Perching stool	It would be unusual for a major kitchen adaptation to be undertaken for a person with a rheumatic condition
Carrying	Continuous worktops and limited distances between key work areas	Wide range of small devices, e.g. trolley, cooking baskets	
Lifting	Consideration of weight of household appliances, e.g. irons, and products, e.g. saucepans		
Reduced reach	Organisation of cupboards, pull out/down shelving in units	Wide range of small devices, e.g. helping hand, cleaning products with extended handles	
Bending	Plug sockets at relevant height		
Grip	Attention to controls on appliances	Large handled plugs	

Table 10.7   Mobility and other activities.

Activity limitation	Mainstream design	Assistive technology	Housing adaptation
Mobility	Intercom	Small mobility aids Manual wheelchair Powered scooter or wheelchair	Intercom
Steps and stairs		Additional rails	Stairlift Ramped access
Communication	Large button phones Use of Skype with headset Ergonomic computer keyboard Voice-activated computer software	Non-slip grips for pens	

needs of older people and people with activity limitations into the design of their products and services have a commercial advantage.

The growth of inclusive design has significant implications for people with rheumatic conditions: as more companies adopt this approach to design, individual needs are being met by mainstream products, the built environment and services such as transport systems reducing the requirement for bespoke AT solutions and environmental adaptation. As people with rheumatic conditions purchase new household appliances or undertake refurbishment of their kitchen or bathroom, careful consideration of the products they purchase and the design and layout of home environments can reduce the level of activity limitation they experience. Occupational therapists have a key role to play in enabling people with rheumatic conditions to make informed decisions about how best to accommodate their needs within mainstream products.

Inclusive design: products

A relevant example of the success of inclusive design is that of Oxo Good Grips, which was launched in 1990 by Sam Farber whose approach to design was informed by problems his wife encountered in finding products to overcome limitations caused by arthritis. The company was launched with 15 products and has now developed a portfolio of more than 850 products with an annual growth rate in sales of 27% between 1991 and 2009 (Oxo Good Grips 2012). Due to an inclusive approach to design, products which overcome the difficulties of weak and painful grip can now be purchased in high-street stores negating the need to purchase specialist and often costly AT.

Inclusive design: built environment

Increasingly, the need to adopt an inclusive design to the built environment is recognised. The transfer of responsibility for the commissioning of many public health services from the NHS to local authorities in England (DoH 2011) acknowledges the role of environmental design in sustaining and promoting health (DoH 2011). In addition, World Health Organisation (WHO 2007) guidance on age-friendly cities highlights the role of housing, transportation, outdoor spaces and buildings in promoting active ageing and reducing social exclusion.

The Lifetime Homes concept (www.lifetimehomes.org.uk), led by the Joseph Rowntree Foundation, aims to meet the changing needs of occupants over the course of their lifetime, minimising the cost of carrying out home adaptations and negating the need to relocate. The Lifetime Homes standard identifies 16 design criteria related to:

- car parking, access and entrances,
- communal stairways and lifts,
- doorways and halls,
- circulation space,
- potential provision of downstairs bedroom,
- the provision of a downstairs toilet with drainage potential for a shower,
- potential for bathroom and toilet adaptation,
- the ability to accommodate a stairlift and a potential site for a through floor lift,
- ease of access to bath, toilet and basin and potential route for ceiling track hoist and
- window specifications, controls, fixtures and fittings.

It is not just the home environment that requires an inclusive approach to design, as increasing numbers of people over 65 are remaining in the workforce due to a number of factors. Myerson (2008) highlights the rise of the pension age to 67 years by 2028; the shortfall in pension funds requiring people to work longer; an increased appreciation of the knowledge skills and expertise of older workers; anti-age and disability discrimination legislation; and better health in later life. As people remain in the workforce for longer, employers, designers and architects will be required increasingly to engage with the configuration of the workplace to meet the needs of the older worker addressing facilities such as lighting, acoustics and ergonomics (Myerson 2008).

10.10 Conclusion

Given the level of activity limitation experienced by people with rheumatic conditions, the use of AT and environmental adaptation is an essential component of maintaining independence in all areas of daily life. Within a changing context of statutory provision and funding, the need for professional assessment by the occupational therapist is essential not only to recommend appropriate AT through statutory supply but to inform the client's private purchase of AT devices and support informed decision making in the purchase of mainstream products. As designers become increasingly aware of the need to use inclusive product design principles, occupational therapists also have the potential to work collaboratively with designers to inform the design of everyday products. Given the high level of abandonment of AT devices, it is essential for occupational therapists to contribute to the evidence base for AT through a better understanding of the key issues that ensure successful AT usage.

Resources

The following organisations provide a wide range of information, publications and resources via their websites with regard to inclusive design:

* The Helen Hamlyn Centre for Design: www.hhc.rca.ac.uk
* The Design Council: www.designcouncil.org.uk
* The Foundation for Lifetime Homes and Neighbourhoods: www.lifetimehomes. org.uk
* The Centre for Universal Design: www.design.ncsu.edu/cud/
* Universal Design Education On Line: www.udeducation.org

The Assistive Technology Alliance (www.at-alliance.org.uk) brings together four UK charities who provide independent advice about AT: The Foundation for Assistive technology; the DLF; Assist UK and Ricability.

The Foundation for Assistive Technology (FAST 2012) (www.fast.org.uk) aims to improve the design and development of AT bringing together users and developers of AT. FAST maintains:

- a database of AT research and development activity in the UK,
- a list of AT-related continuing professional development and
- current job vacancies in the AT sector.

The DLF (http://www.dlf.org.uk/) provides independent advice and information about AT including:

- advisory telephone helpline,
- an independent online database of AT available through a subscription,
- 'Living Made Easy', a web-based information portal,
- Fact sheets about AT for a wide range of daily living tasks,
- 'AskSara' (described previously),
- a London-based demonstration centre and
- a supplier directory.

Assist UK (www.assist-uk.org) leads a network of over 60 local Disabled Living Centres across the UK who provide independent advice and support through permanent exhibition centres employing professional advisory staff.

Ricability (www.ricability.org.uk), a consumer affairs charity, produces independent consumer reports on devices for mobility, personal care, in the home and parenting and consumer rights. Reports are available free of charge and can be downloaded from their website.

References

Ahtola S, Heinonen A, Haikonen K, et al. (2011) Adaptation and validation of the modified KWAZO and EATS-2D instruments into Finnish circumstances. In: Gelderblom GJ, Soede M, Adriaens L, Miesenberger K (eds.) *Everyday Technology for Independence and Care – AAATE 2011 Vol. 29 Assistive Technology Research Series*. Lansdale, PA: IOS Press.

Assist UK and Ricability (2011) *Fit to Equip*? Second year Report prepared for the Department of Health. www.assist-uk.org/images/pdfs/mystery%20shopping%20report%202011.pdf. Accessed on 14 November 2012.

Bougie T (2003) *ICF and ISO9999 to Express Intended Use of Assistive Technology*. Koln: WHO Collaborating Centres.www.interbor.org. Accessed on 14 November 2012.

Clinical Guidelines Working Group, National Association of Rheumatology Occupational Therapists (COT) (2003) *Occupational Therapy Clinical Guidelines for Rheumatology*. London: College of Occupational Therapists.

Coleman R (2006) *From Margins to Mainstream. Why Inclusive Design Matter*. London: Helen Hamlyn Research Centre London. http://www.hhc.rca.ac.uk/CMS/files/ErgSocLecture06.pdf. Accessed on 10 March 2012.

Cook A, Hussey S (2002) *Assistive Technologies: Principles and Practice* (2nd edn.). St. Louis, MO: Mosby Inc.

Cowan D, Turner-Smith A (1991) *The Role of Assistive Technology in Alternative Models of Care for Older People. With Respect to Old Age – Research*, Vol. 2. London: Her Majesty's Stationary Office.

Day H, Jutai J (1996) *Psychosocial Impact of Assistive Devices Scale*. http://www.piads.net/9/index1.2.html. Accessed on 10 March 2012.

de Boer I, Peeters A, Ronday H, et al. (2009) Assistive devices: Usage in patients with rheumatoid arthritis. *Clinical Rheumatology* 28:119–128.

Demers L, Monette M, Lapierre Y, et al. (2002a) Reliability, validity, and applicability of the Quebec User Evaluation of Satisfaction with assistive Technology (QUEST2.0) for adults with multiple Sclerosis. *Disability and Rehabilitation* 24(1):21–30.

Demers L, Weiss Lambrou R, Ska B (2002b) The Quebec Evaluation of satisfaction with Assistive technology (QUEST 2.0): An overview with recent progress. *Technology and Disability* 14:101–105.

Department of Health (DoH) (2011) *The New Public Health System: Summary*. London: DoH. http://www.dh.gov.uk/prod_consum_dh/groups/dh_digitalassets/documents/digitalasset/dh_131897.pdf. Accessed on 10 March 2012.

Design Council Living Longer (2012). http://www.designcouncil.org.uk/publications/living-longer/. Accessed on 10 February 2012.

Dijcks P, Wessels R, De Vlieger S, et al. (2006) KWAZO, a new instrument to assess the quality of service delivery in assistive technology provision. *Disability and Rehabilitation* 28(15):909–914.

Foundation for Assistive Technology (2012) *Definition of Assistive Technology*. http://www.fastuk.org/about/definitionofat.php. Accessed on 14 November 2012.

Giesbrecht E, Ripat J, Quanbury A, et al. (2009) Participation in community-based activities of daily living: Comparison of a pushrim-activated, power-assisted wheelchair and a power wheelchair. *Disability and Rehabilitation: Assistive Technology* 4(3):198–207.

Goodacre L, Turner G (2005) The use of the Quebec User Evaluation of Satisfaction with assistive Technology for adults supplied with Stairlifts. *British Journal of Occupational Therapy* 68(2):93–96.

Hammond A (2004) What is the role of the occupational therapist? Best practice and research. *Clinical Rheumatology* 18(4):491–505.

Hocking C (1999) Function or feelings: Factors in abandonment of assistive devices. *Technology and Disability* 11(1,2):3.

Karlsson P (2003) *ICF: A Guide to Assistive Technology Decision-Making*. www.arata.org.au/arataconf10/papers/KARLSSON_Petra_paper_arata10.doc. Accessed on 10 March 2012.

Myerson J (2008) *Welcoming Workspaces. Designing Office Space for an Ageing Workforce in the 21st Century Knowledge Economy. A Guide for Architects and Developers*. London: Helen Hamlyn Centre, Royal College of Art. http://www.hhc.rca.ac.uk/462/all/1/publications.aspx. Accessed on 10 March 2012.

Office of the Deputy Prime Minister (2005) *Improving the Life Chances of Disabled People*. http://www.dh.gov.uk/en/Publicationsandstatistics/Publications/PublicationsPolicyAndGuidance/DH_4101751. Accessed on 10 March 2012.

Oxo Good Grips (2012) *Universal Design*. http://www.oxo.com/UniversalDesign.aspx. Accessed on 10 March 2012.

Petty L, McArthur L, Treviranus J, et al. (2005) Clinical report: Use of the Canadian Occupational Performance Measure in vision technology. *Canadian Journal of Occupational Therapy* 72(5):309–312.

Ripat J (2006) Function and impact of electronic aids to daily living for experienced users. *Technology & Disability* 18(2):79–87.

Ripat J, Booth A (2005) Characteristics of assistive technology service delivery models: Stakeholder perspectives and preferences. *Disability and Rehabilitation* 27(24):1461–1470.

Scherer MJ (2000) *Living in the State of Stuck: How Assistive Technology Impacts the Lives of People with Disabilities.* Cambridge, MA: Brookline Books Inc.

Scherer MJ, Sax C, Vanbiervliet A, et al. (2005) Predictors of assistive technology use: The importance of personal and psychosocial factors. *Disability and Rehabilitation* 27(21):1321–1331.

Tuntland H, Kjeken I, Nordheim L, et al. (2009) Assistive technology for rheumatoid arthritis. *Cochrane Database of Systematic Reviews* 4:CD006729.

Vanderheiden CG (1991) Service delivery mechanisms in rehabilitation technology. *American Journal of Occupational Therapy* 41:703–710.

Wessels R, Dijcks B, Soede M, et al. (2003) Non-use of provided assistive technology devices, a literature overview. *Technology and Disability* 15:231–238.

Wessels R, De Witte L, Van den Heuvel W (2004) Measuring effectiveness of and satisfaction with assistive devices from a user perspective: An exploration of the literature. *Technology & Disability* 16(2):83–90.

Winchcombe M, Ballinger C (2005) A *Competence Framework for Trusted Assessors*. London: Assist UK. http://www.cot.co.uk/sites/default/files/publications/public/Competence-framework.pdf. Accessed on 10 March 2012.

World Health Organisation (WHO) (2001) International Classification of Functioning, Disability and Health (ICF). Geneva, Switzerland: WHO. http://www.who.int/classifications/icf/en. Accessed on 25 March 2012.

WHO (2004) *Glossary of Terms for Community Health Care and Services for Older Persons.* Geneva, Switzerland: WHO.

WHO (2007) *Global Age Friendly Cities.* Geneva, Switzerland: WHO.

Chapter 11

Vocational rehabilitation

Lucy Reeve[1] and Janet Harkess[2]

[1]*Rheumatology Department, Norfolk and Norwich University Hospital, Norwich, United Kingdom;*
[2]*Fife Rheumatic Diseases Unit, Fife, Scotland*

11.1 Introduction

Rheumatic conditions affect the lives of individuals in many ways, one of the most important of which is work disability (WD). In the UK, many people with rheumatic conditions lose their jobs early in the disease process, even before being referred to hospital or starting treatment (Baker and Pope 2009; Barlow 2009; Barrett et al. 2000).

Participation in work is not a simple dichotomy of working versus not working. Research indicates that prior to job loss people experience the stress of work limitations and potential changes to their existing jobs or changes of career to maintain employment. People reduce their working hours, miss out on promotion opportunities and experience increased sick leave or change jobs with greater frequency before taking early retirement on health grounds (Backman 2004; Gignac et al. 2008). As a consequence, under-employment, reduction of income and decreased job satisfaction are common (Allaire 1998; Kim et al. 2001).

> *Work disability* – The inability to continue working, to work in the same occupation or to work the same number of hours
> *Vocational rehabilitation* – A process to overcome the barriers an individual faces as a result of injury, illness or impairment when accessing, remaining in or returning to purposeful activity, work and employment (COT 2008).

There are a number of issues associated with rheumatic conditions that influence peoples' working lives. Firstly, for those in work unpredictable exacerbations and

Rheumatology Practice in Occupational Therapy: Promoting Lifestyle Management, First Edition.
Edited by Lynne Goodacre and Margaret McArthur.
© 2013 John Wiley & Sons, Ltd. Published 2013 by John Wiley & Sons, Ltd.

remission create difficulties with predicting and planning work activities. Systemic symptoms may reduce working ability and lead to inconsistent levels of performance. These problems are compounded in settings where people have little control over the pace and type of work activities, often leading to people working beyond their physical capabilities. With symptoms such as morning stiffness and functional limitations, the challenges begin *before* work, necessitating an earlier start to the day. Those considering partial return to work can become fearful about the impact of working on their physical and financial well-being. Lastly, for those out of work fluctuating disease interferes with the ability to consistently seek work and maintain work skills (McArthur 2002).

11.2   The importance of employment

Occupational therapists acknowledge that work plays a significant role in shaping the daily pattern of peoples' lives and is important for the maintenance of self-esteem, personal identity and status in society. Some people see work as an instrument to achieving a particular end, such as providing an income to maintain their living standards. For others work gives a sense of value and enjoyment providing social contacts, a context in which to perform meaningful activities, an arena for personal growth and achievement (Persson et al. 2011) and a means of retaining independence and earning money (Barlow et al. 2001).

When the onset of a rheumatic condition occurs early in a working life, it can have profound effects on the individual and their family, particularly due to loss of earnings and ability to accumulate assets for retirement. Therefore, most people want to continue working (Henriksson et al. 2005). Furthermore, work can be beneficial to health (Waddell and Burton 2006), e.g., involvement in interesting tasks can bring temporary distraction from pain and discomfort (Jakobsen 2001). Conversely unemployment is associated with poorer health, increased long-term conditions and increased mortality (Gerdtham and Johannesson 2003; Mathers and Schofield 1998).

11.3   The current context of vocational rehabilitation

Informed by the Black Report (Black 2008) government policy currently focuses on ensuring that everyone with the potential to work has the support they need to do so. Whilst the labour market and the political backdrop that influences it are ever-changing, there is a commitment to increasing the number of people with disabilities in the workforce, which has been brought about through the Disability Discrimination Acts (DDA) (1995, 2005) and the Equality Act (2010). Alongside legislation, various Welfare to Work schemes have been introduced to facilitate employment for those with disabilities by focusing on what people *can do* instead of what they cannot, adopting a more flexible and constructive approach to help people to return to work more successfully (Black 2008).

11.4 Predictors of work disability and work instability

The effectiveness of any therapeutic interventions (clinical or vocational) requires an understanding of potential factors that can affect the work situation. There are a range of potentially influential factors and considerable variation in peoples' employment experiences; however, the actual combination of factors and their relative importance in predicting WD or work-related changes remain unclear (Lacaille 2007). Risk factors for WD are present at both an individual and a societal level. The most common fall into three categories.

Disease characteristics

Rheumatic conditions are chronic and unpredictable, with ongoing pain and inflammation, and systemic symptoms, such as fatigue, usually imposing functional limitations affecting daily activities, ability to work and quality of life (Dubouloz et al. 2008). However, the influence of disease characteristics on employment remains controversial. In a systematic review of RA and WD, physical job demands, low functional capacity, old age and low education were the only consistent factors to predict WD whilst biomedical variables did not (De Croon 2004). Other research suggests that a high erythrocyte sedimentation rate, greater pain/fatigue scores, disease duration, structural damage and limited functional disability *are* associated with WD (Baker and Pope 2009; Sokka et al. 2010). However, more importantly, clients consistently report that pain, physical limitations, fatigue, morning stiffness and having to take time off sick are the main barriers to employment (Lacaille 2007; Westhoff et al. 2008). Interestingly, people with comparable levels of disease activity may differ greatly in their work capacity, indicating that social and work-related factors may have a greater impact on WD than biomedical factors (Yelin et al. 1987).

The impact of medication in reducing WD also remains unclear. Some studies indicate that work loss occurs despite medical intervention (Allaire et al. 2008; Filipovic et al. 2011), whereas others suggest that early aggressive intervention may impact on the course of the rheumatic condition and improve a person's ability to maintain employment (Boers 2003; Puolakka et al. 2004). However, clients report that accommodating treatment demands can be difficult within many work settings. The healthcare system does not assist people in employment, as clinics are usually held during the day, necessitating time off work (Barlow 2009).

Job characteristics

The 'right job' (including the physical, cognitive and psychological demands) with the 'right support' in the 'right environment' facilitates maintenance of employment (Frank and Thurgood 2006; Ross 2008). For example, repetitive and heavy tasks or those requiring prolonged standing or sitting are particularly problematic (Geuskens et al. 2008; Mancuso et al. 2000). Those able to control the pace of work or who are self-employed are more likely to continue working (Yelin et al. 1980, 1987), for instance, being able to start later in the morning to take account of morning stiffness, adjusting the pace of work activities, leaving early or taking time off to accommodate pain or a 'flare' (Newman et al. 1996).

A positive work environment where both employer and colleagues have an understanding of a person's condition and appreciate the contribution they make were consistently identified as important to maintaining employment. Many problems associated with work have been identified as being manageable if colleagues and employers understand, are prepared to offer practical assistance and be flexible (Henriksson et al. 2005; NRAS 2007). From the employer's perspective the size of the company, availability of modified duties and return to work policies are influential (Ross 2008). Environmental barriers frequently arise from the inappropriate design of buildings, including access to facilities such as toilets and parking, layout of the workstation and nature of any equipment used (Frank and Thurgood 2006), as well as transport difficulties (Barlow 2009).

Socio-demographic variables

Advancing age, lower educational level and being female are associated with WD, whereas being married, having family support and higher socioeconomic status appear to be protective factors (Baker and Pope 2009; De Croon 2004; Filipovic et al. 2011). However, such research has little clinical utility as these factors cannot be readily changed. It is therefore more important to focus on what people can do to change their circumstances in order to enter the workplace or maintain their position in it (Yeung 2010).

People also face a number of barriers at a societal level including lack of understanding about rheumatic conditions and the invisible or fluctuating nature of symptoms; the unemployment rate and local work opportunities; laws and regulations regarding work; and benefits and pension plans (Barlow 2009).

Furthermore, people with rheumatic conditions can be challenged by the expectations of an achievement-orientated society, especially men who are more likely to prioritise paid work commitments over their health concerns. It still appears to be more acceptable for women to opt out of the workforce (Stamm et al. 2010). Work is significantly influenced by the personal meaning attached to it. So, a person's knowledge regarding their illness, their previous experiences, their attitudes and beliefs about work and illness as well as their pre-disease perceptions of self contribute to their decision to withdraw or remain in work (Shaw et al. 2006).

11.5 Vocational rehabilitation

At present, there is a lack of robust evidence that vocational rehabilitation (VR) for people with rheumatic conditions is effective, which is disappointing as people report finding work assessment and interventions particularly beneficial (NICE 2009;

Steutjens et al. 2008). Evidence from a systematic review of VR found that a team approach to VR was the most effective way to reduce WD (De Buck et al. 2005) and Macedo et al. (2009) demonstrated that comprehensive occupational therapy improved functional and work outcomes.

Unfortunately, difficulties with work are often not sufficiently acknowledged by healthcare professionals (NICE 2009, p. 61; Varekamp et al. 2005), and it seems that the majority of people have to negotiate their own workplace adaptations and modes of working (Barlow 2009). Among younger people, the focus is on encouraging attempts to enter the labour market, but it appears that few young people with arthritis receive adequate vocational guidance or counselling, with lack of awareness, confidence and support being sighted as barriers to employment (Straughair and Fawcit 1992). Shaw et al. (2006) identified that vocational support for adolescents with inflammatory arthrtides remains uncoordinated, limited and unresponsive to individual needs.

11.6 Occupational therapy and vocational rehabilitation

Occupational therapists are key players in VR being involved in the assessment, treatment and coordination of work issues as outlined in the COT VR Strategy (COT 2008). The nature and extent of the occupational therapy role for people with rheumatic conditions varies considerably between clients, but broadly comes under two categories: *work-specific interventions* such as worksite assessments and meetings with employers, and *condition-specific interventions* such as joint protection advice, pain and fatigue management.

Timing of interventions

Prevention of WD is an important treatment goal, especially when onset of the rheumatic condition is at a relatively early age and when the impact on lifestyle, career path, family and social life could be long term and far reaching (Barlow 2009). Therefore, a careful analysis of their work, workplace, work commitments and future plans and aspirations is required as early as possible after onset of the condition (Eberhardt 2009). However, the timing of such interventions needs to be evaluated on an individual basis. Significant changes to the work situation, such as changing job or career, cannot be decided until the person has begun to accept that their life has changed as a result of their condition and that adjustments are necessary (Henriksson et al. 2005).

Work assessment

Work assessment is most effective when it is an integral part of a wider holistic appreciation of the impact someone's health condition has in all areas of their life (Gilworth et al. 2003). Symptoms not only impact on work but also on everyday activities at home; therefore, people have to find solutions to everyday challenges and make adaptations in all areas to facilitate their employment activities (Jakobsen 2001). Work is only one of the occupational roles that people hold and the decisions they make about employment are influenced by their total life situation (Shaw et al. 2006). For example, domestic and childcare duties also demand time and energy from someone with potentially limited capacity.

Work interview and job analysis

A detailed assessment of a person's work situation and how their impairment affects their ability to work is essential for effective VR (Joss 2007). An initial work interview should gather as much information as possible about the person and their job to highlight areas of concern. Asking the question 'Are you having any problems at work?' usually leads to a discussion regarding the nature of their work and the tasks involved. This may be accompanied by a more detailed assessment of the physical working conditions; work activities throughout the day, typical daily routine, tasks involved, breaks and level of control over that routine; the person's functional abilities and work tolerance; transportation to work; interpersonal relationships at work; and lastly sources of stress (Melvin and Jensen 1998). Additional information may include:

- Current medication and other therapies.
- Specific joint symptoms, fatigue/pain visual analogue scale (VAS) and any other medical issues affecting work performance.
- Abilities, roles and routines at home and within leisure areas.
- Educational background.
- Past employment history and occupational interests/aptitudes.
- Current employment details (job title, employer's details, hours of work, shift pattern, previous and current sick leave).
- Financial status.
- Details of occupational health provider and their involvement.
- Psychosocial information – job importance and satisfaction, perceived stress.
- Job demands – main components of the job.
- Job concerns – specific work-related problems in order of importance.
- Actions already taken to try and address work issues.

Worksite assessment

A worksite assessment can enable the therapist to observe at first hand the demands of someone's job and carry out ergonomic analysis of the work environment. This may also provide insights into the interpersonal dynamics. Such assessments require permission from the client (and employer) and should ideally be organised by the client. Suggestions about the type of information the occupational therapist may collect include:

1 Physical demands, e.g. sitting, standing, walking, manual dexterity, manual handling.
2 Environmental demands, e.g. indoor or outdoor, temperature, vibration.
3 Access:
   ○ External environment – e.g. parking, public transport.
   ○ Internal environment – e.g. lifts, steps, doors.
   ○ Facilities – e.g. catering, rest areas.
4 Equipment used.

11.7   Work evaluation and monitoring

Appropriate screening tools and assessments provide an accurate knowledge base for treatment planning and a baseline for subsequent evaluation of interventions. There are a variety of work-specific assessment tools (COT 2008) including the Rheumatoid Arthritis Work Instability Scale (RA-WIS) and the Ankylosing Spondylitis Work Instability Scale (AS-WIS) (Gilworth et al. 2003). These self-administered questionnaires classify the level of work instability as low, medium and high and help identify those at most risk and in need of intervention. They can be used for initial screening, monitoring of work circumstances and as outcome measures (Macedo et al. 2009). Work by Allaire and Keysor (2009) and Osterhaus et al. (2009) may provide further RD-specific work assessment in the future.

Other tools include:

* The Canadian Occupational Performance Measure (COPM) (Law et al. 1998).
* The Health Assessment Questionnaire (Fries et al. 1980), which in research into RA and WD was the most important predictor of WD (Young et al. 2002) and has been used to measure the effects of occupational therapy on functional and work outcomes (Macedo et al. 2009).
* Levels of satisfaction and work performance assessed using a 10 cm visual analogue scale.
* The amount of sick leave taken, which in people in the early stages of their rheumatic condition appears to be a significant factor in predicting WD (Zirkzee et al. 2008).

Due to the variability of rheumatic conditions and peoples' life circumstances and employment naturally changing over time, there is a need for employment-related issues to be addressed on an ongoing basis. Current evidence supports the use of early interventions to maintain people in employment (Eberhardt 2009), as it is easier to keep people in work than try and get them back to work once they have been out of work for some time (Gilworth et al. 2003). Needs-led access to the rheumatology team was identified in a National Rheumatoid Arthritis Society survey (2007) by over half of all respondents as the most important measure thought to enable them to remain in employment. It is also important to evaluate work interventions by audit and regular service review (Harkess 2010).

11.8   Condition-specific interventions

Fray (2008) maintains that managing arthritis is crucial to managing at work; therefore, effective work interventions will facilitate clients' management of symptoms such as pain and fatigue. Such interventions include education; joint protection and lifestyle management advice; the provision of orthoses; and assistive equipment (Hammond et al. 2008; Hewlett et al. 2011; Steutjens et al. 2008) (Box 11.1).

11.9   Work-specific interventions

The type of vocational support and advice will vary considerably between clients. For some people, verbal or written advice may be appropriate whilst others may require more complex interventions.

Job modification

The aim of job modification is to match the job and the person supported by the legal requirement for the employer to make 'reasonable adjustments' under the 2010 Equality Act (Box 11.2). Flexibility is particularly necessary for people with variable symptoms and those with significant early morning stiffness, regular flares and fatigue (Henriksson et al. 2005). This may include temporary or permanent changes to start and finish times, hours, or days; the protection or establishment of regular breaks; as well as changes of task and work task positions. Flexibility may also involve task modification such as doing the task in a different way, altering the duties in someone's

---

Box 11.1   Condition management case study

Mike is 45 years old, has Systemic Lupus Erythematosus and is an area manager for a plant hire firm. His job involved extended hours of work, a lot of travel and he had poor sleep hygiene. Occupational therapy assessment found that Mike scored:

• Fatigue – 8/10 VAS.
• COPM – work performance 6/10; work satisfaction 5/10.

Mike had fatigue management training encompassing:

• Pacing – included avoiding overtime where possible.
• Planning – involved staying away overnight once a week and using train and taxis instead of the car where possible.
• He was also directed to Access to Work for financial assistance with additional travel costs.
• Sleep hygiene advice included reducing caffeine intake.

On review Mike had implemented all of the suggestions. Re-assessment highlighted improved scores of:

• Fatigue – 6/10 VAS.
• COPM – work performance 8/10; work satisfaction 8/10.

Box 11.2   Job modification case study

David is 53 years old, has Ankylosing Spondylitis and works as an engineer in a factory on a shift work pattern. His work difficulties included:

- Pain – 8/10 VAS.
- Fatigue – 7/10 VAS.
- Reduced prehensile grip.
- AS-WIS score indicated high work instability at 17/20.
- COPM – work performance 5/10; work satisfaction 5/10.

An occupational therapy work site assessment resulted in a recommendation of lighter duties and if possible just day time shifts. The company was unable to modify David's current job but offered him an alternative job in the office with regular day time hours. This involved a slight pay cut and some additional training on IT systems but David accepted this offer.

On review David was much improved and scored:

- Pain – 5/10 VAS.
- Fatigue – 5/10 VAS.
- AS-WIS – low work instability at 10/20.
- COPM – 9/10 for work performance; 8/10 for satisfaction.

job description, job sharing, exchange or delegation of certain tasks to others. Additional training to facilitate redeployment would also be classified as reasonable adjustment. Employees may also negotiate time for hospital appointments and home working. Any job modifications should consider someone's present and future economic situation to fully calculate the consequences of interventions. For example, pension and benefits may be affected if the person reduces their working hours.

Environmental adaptation

Ergonomic principles are commonly used in the work environment to enable tasks to be carried out as efficiently as possible, with minimum stress on the joints and to reduce pain and fatigue in accordance with the principles of joint protection and energy conservation (Melvin and Jensen 1998). Modification of the environment may involve adaptations to the workplace or person's workstation, e.g. provision of an ergonomic chair or keyboard, changing the layout or position of the workstation or improving access to toilets or parking. This type of intervention is currently supported by the Access to Work Scheme (Department of Work and Pensions 2012).

Return to work

Return to work planning usually includes an assessment of someone's work readiness and fitness to work and may involve working with the person and their employer to devise a suitable plan for returning to work in accordance with their current health situation (Box 11.3). The therapist may provide an informal letter with recommendations for reasonable adjustments or a formal report detailing a return to work plan that outlines days and hours to be worked with recommended incremental alterations to

> **Box 11.3   Return to work case study**
>
> Susan is 36 years old, has Rheumatoid Arthritis and has been receiving employment support allowance for 4 years. An occupational therapy assessment identified that Susan had previous experience working as a receptionist; that Susan's IT skills needed updating but she was physically able to try a sedentary/light job. With occupational therapy support Susan:
>
> - updated her computer skills
> - got advice from a local employment agency on completing job applications and updating her CV
> - accessed occupational therapy support by telephone
>
> Susan got a part time job as a receptionist at the local swimming pool. A workstation ergonomic review found that no modifications were required. A telephone occupational therapy review consultation at 1 month highlighted:
>
> - a low RA-WIS of 9/23
>
> A review 4 months later highlighted:
>
> - a lower RA-WIS of 4/23

tasks and environmental adjustments. A well-planned return to work allows the employee to build up stamina and confidence in the work situation (Ross 2008).

Work preparation and hardening may be appropriate for some clients dependent on the resources available to the therapist. Alternatively, advice may be given about activities that can be carried out at home to build up stamina and abilities (Gibson et al. 2002; Melvin and Jensen 1998).

11.10   Advice on redeployment or retraining

Sometimes, redeployment or retraining has to be considered particularly if a job would require impractical or unreasonable modification or because of health and safety concerns. In these circumstances, the person may need to be assessed for deployment, retraining or medical retirement. Those people who want or need to continue within another form of employment can be referred to local employment agencies for support. Therapists can help them identify existing skills and educational achievements or future training needs and suitable career choices. Local adult education and employment agencies can help with job applications, CV and interview techniques. They may also provide information on potential financial support.

11.11   Counselling and advocacy

Many people who are seemingly successfully employed face substantial difficulties and considerable stress to maintain their jobs (Mancuso et al. 2000). People experience pressure to demonstrate their competence and fulfil the expectation of others in spite of their illness; many are often exhausted after a day's work, leaving little energy for home and family activities (Jakobsen 2001). Anxiety about having time off and the future is common and appears to manifest as guilt and a feeling of vulnerability in terms of job security (Barlow 2009; Mancuso et al. 2000).

Issues of disclosure or concealment of their disability and accompanying functional limitations can be a real concern for some people, who may try to conceal pain or difficulties they experience believing that revealing a disability may result in them being categorised as helpless or incompetent. Others find that there is a very fine dividing line between obtaining necessary help and unwanted attention (Allen and Carlson 2003).

Work instability has been associated with higher levels of pain and depression (Fifield et al. 2004), and depression was associated with work changes such as occasional work loss and changes in type/hours of work (Gignac et al. 2004). Whether depression is related to the impact of a health condition or specifically related to employment changes is not clear. However, identity is often linked to work and feelings of independence, and so loss of work or changes in role could potentially result in feelings of depression and lower self-esteem (Jakobsen 2001). A young woman with scleroderma, when describing the impact her condition had on her ability to work, explained that:

> I had always worked full time, earning a good wage with respect from my colleagues. I had my career progression mapped out, and then my health got worse. Some days I hardly knew what to do with myself. I was exhausted. My joints hurt and I couldn't do what I wanted no matter how hard I tried.

She tried to accommodate the changes in her health 'I changed my job. I decreased my hours once, then again'; however, such changes had a devastating impact on her identity and emotions, 'I felt like I was failing and hopeless. I lost my identity and sense of competence and confidence'.

Loss of confidence and reduced self-esteem may lead people to believe that they have little to offer and therefore cease attempts to enter or remain in the employment market (Barlow 2009). Therefore, an important aspect of the occupational therapist's role is the provision of counselling and support. Empowering people through the use of stress management, assertiveness and communication skills training may be valuable interventions (Allen and Carlson 2003; Macedo et al. 2009). This includes teaching problem-solving skills to enable people to develop a solution-focused approach to the barriers they face in work.

Therapists can also assume an advocacy role through liaison with the employer and appropriate others to help people navigate the employment and welfare services. This would include supporting someone to disclose their disability, educate their employer and colleagues about their condition and negotiate any reasonable adjustments at work.

11.12 Post-work support

For many people with disabilities, becoming unemployed is a major transition which involves much more than a loss of income. The decision to leave work is a stressful time in someone's life necessitating a reappraisal of self-concept and roles. Many people report a diminished sense of self and personal autonomy and interpret loss of work as evidence of personal failure and inadequacy, and they lose traction within their life trajectory (McArthur 2002).

Although the meaning of work varies with individual circumstances, those unable to work are faced with finding alternative activities to fill their time. Occupational therapy can provide an opportunity to exploring alternative meaningful activities facilitated both through the initial interview and using tools such as the MOHO related UK Modified Interest Checklist (Heasman and Brewer 2008).

11.13 Summary

For some people, effective therapeutic intervention means that their symptoms are greatly improved leading to improvement in their work functioning. However, it is clear that many people continue to face challenges in their working life and for others employment is not sustainable (Filipovic et al. 2011). Therefore, therapists need to consistently ask about work so they can provide timely and appropriate support and advice. This should involve a multi-faceted approach to work assessment to identify and deal with the complex array of factors which influence the working lives of people with rheumatic conditions. Ultimately, the extent to which these problems can be managed or solved determines whether someone can remain in work (Ross 2008).

People with rheumatic conditions have to negotiate numerous areas of their life in order to be successfully employed. However, when people find a level that matches their ability, they can continue to work and find satisfaction in their work role. Maintaining employment can be viewed as a developmental process rather than a one-off event requiring the person to develop the personal skills and flexibility needed to deal with current and future issues (Jakobsen 2001; Roessler et al. 1998).

Current evidence supports the use of early interventions (Eberhardt 2009) as it is easier to keep people in work than try to get them back to work (Gilworth et al. 2003). Therefore, employment issues should be highlighted at diagnosis.

There is a two-way relationship between illness and work, and for some people work may have a detrimental impact on their health (Codd et al. 2010; Fifield et al. 2004) due to the significant adaptations some people make in their personal lives to continue working which may be detrimental to their quality of life (Allaire 1998; Jakobsen 2001). Reliance on family members, modification of the home routine and reducing family and social activities are common (Mancuso et al. 2000; NRAS 2007). Therefore, it is not surprising that some people view stopping work positively as they may have the time, energy and opportunity to achieve a better occupational balance, improved health and quality of life (Stamm et al. 2004). Therapists need to recognise the costs *as well as* the benefits of working to help people to make a balanced decision about changes they make to employment.

Resources

Ability Net: Provides Advice on Computing and Disability. http://www.abilitynet.org.uk. Accessed on 14 November 2012.

Arthritis Care: Working With Arthritis (3rd edn.). London: Arthritis Care. http://www.arthritiscare. org.uk/PublicationsandResources/Listedbytype/Booklets. Accessed on 14 November 2012.

Arthritis Research UK (ARUK): Work and Arthritis Leaflet.
http://www.arthritisresearchuk.org/arthritis-information/arthritis-and-daily-life/work-and-arthritis.aspx. Accessed on 14 November 2012.

College of Occupational Therapists – 'Work Matters'. http://www.cot.co.uk/sites/default/files/ publications/public/work-matters-final-11.07.pdf. Accessed on 16 March 2012.

Directgov – Information on employment support for people with disabilities including looking for work, work schemes, support while in work and employment rights. http://www.direct. gov.uk/en/DisabledPeople/Employmentsupport/index.htm. Accessed on 14 November 2012.

Disabled Workers Co-operative: Aims to help people with disabilities by enabling them to take an active role in the economy and achieve a greater sense of self-worth. http://www. disabledworkers.org.uk/. Accessed on 14 November 2012.

Employers' Forum on Disability: An employers' organisation focused on disability aiming to facilitate the recruitment and retention of employees with disabilities. http://www.efd.org.uk/. Accessed on 14 November 2012.

LearnDirect: An e-learning organisation set up by University for Industry. http://learndirect. co.uk/. Accessed on 14 November 2012.

National Institute for Clinical and Heath Excellence (NICE) – *NICE Guideline for the Management of Long-Term Sickness and Incapacity for Work.* http://guidance.nice.org.uk/ PH19/Guidance/pdf/English Accessed on 14 November 2012.

National Rheumatoid Arthritis Society: *'I Want To Work – A Self Help Guide For People With Rheumatoid Arthritis'* and *'When An Employee Has Rheumatoid Arthritis – An Employer's Guide'*. www.nras.org.uk. Accessed on 14 November 2012.

Shaw Trust: Supports people to prepare for work, find jobs and live more independently. http://www.shaw-trust.org.uk/home. Accessed on 14 November 2012.

Worker Role Interview: Velozo C, Keilhofner G, Fisher G (1998) *A Users Guide to Worker Role Interview (WRI), Version 9.0.* Model of Human Occupation, Clearing House, USA. Chicago, IL: University of Illinois.

Worklife: Advice and support for clients, employers and healthcare professionals. http://www. yourworkhealth.com/. Accessed on 14 November 2012.

WorkWise: Workshop presentation summaries and helpful contacts.
www.nras.org.uk/includes/documents/cm_docs/2011/p/patient_booklet.pdf. Accessed on 14 November 2012.

References

Allaire SH (1998) Vocational rehabilitation for persons with rheumatoid arthritis. *Journal of Vocational Rehabilitation* 10:253–260.

Allaire S, Keysor JJ (2009) Development of a structured interview tool to help clients identify and solve rheumatic condition-related work barriers. *Arthritis Care & Research* 61(7):988–995.

Allaire S, Wolfe F, Niu J, et al. (2008) Contemporary prevalence and incidence of work disability associated with rheumatoid arthritis in the US. *Arthritis Care & Research* 34(11):2211–2217.

Allen S, Carlson G (2003) To conceal or disclose a disabling condition? A dilemma of employment transition. *Journal of Vocational Rehabilitation* 19:19–30.

Backman C (2004) Employment and work disability in rheumatoid arthritis. *Current Opinion in Rheumatology* 16:148–152.

Baker K, Pope J (2009) Employment and work disability in systemic lupus erthematosus: A systematic review. *Rheumatology* 48(3):281–284.

Barlow J (2009) *Living with Arthritis*. Oxford, UK: The British Psychological Society, Blackwell.

Barlow J, Wright C, Krol T (2001) Overcoming perceived barriers to employment among people with arthritis. *Journal of Health Psychology* 6(2):205–216.

Barrett E, Scott D, Wiles N, et al. (2000) The impact of rheumatoid arthritis on employment status in the early years of disease: A UK community based study. *Rheumatology* 39(12):1403–1409.

Black D (2008) *Working for a Healthier Tomorrow*. London: The Stationary Office.

Boers M (2003) Understanding the window of opportunity concept in early rheumatoid arthritis. *Arthritis & Rheumatism* 48:1771–1774.

Codd Y, Stapleton T, Veale D, et al. (2010) A qualitative study of work participation in early rheumatoid arthritis. *International Journal of Therapy and Rehabilitation* 17(1):24–33.

College of Occupational Therapists (COT) (2008) *The College of Occupational Therapists Vocational Rehabilitation Strategy*. London: COT.

De Buck P, Le Cessie S, Van Den Hout, et al. (2005) Randomised comparison of a multidisciplinary job-retention vocational rehabilitation program with usual outpatient care in patients with chronic arthritis at risk for job loss. *Arthritis Care and Research* 53(5): 682–690.

De Croon EM (2004) Predictive factors of work disability in rheumatoid arthritis: A systematic literature review. *Annals of the Rheumatic Diseases* 63(11):1362–1367.

Department of Work and Pensions (2012) *Access to Work Scheme*. http://www.direct.gov.uk/en/DisabledPeople/Employmentsupport/WorkSchemesAndProgrammes/DG_4000347. Accessed on 17 March 2012.

Disability Discrimination Act (1995) http://www.legislation.gov.uk/ukpga/1995/50/contents. Accessed on 14 November 2012.

Disability Discrimination Act (2005) http://www.legislation.gov.uk/ukpga/2005/13/contents. Accessed on 14 November 2012.

Dubouloz CJ, Vallerand J, Laporte D, et al. (2008) Occupational performance modification and personal change among clients receiving rehabilitation services for rheumatoid arthritis. *Australian Occupational Therapy Journal* 55:30–38.

Eberhardt K (2009) Editorial: Very early intervention is crucial to improve work outcome in patients with rheumatoid arthritis. *The Journal of Rheumatology* 36:6.

Equality Act (2010) http://homeoffice.gov.uk/equalities/equality-act/index.html. Accessed 19 November 2012.

Fifield J, McQuillan J, Armeli S, et al. (2004) Chronic strain, daily work stress and pain among workers with rheumatoid arthritis: Does job stress make a bad day worse? *Work and Stress* 18(4):275–291.

Filipovic I, Walker D, Forster F, et al. (2011) Quantifying the economic burden of productivity loss in rheumatoid arthritis. *Rheumatology* 50:1083–1090.

Frank AO, Thurgood J (2006) Vocational rehabilitation in the UK: Opportunities for health care professionals. *International Journal of Therapy and Rehabilitation* 13(3):126–134.

Fray L (2008) A working life. *Arthritis News* Oct/Nov.

Fries JF, Spitz P, Kraines RG (1980) Measurement of patient outcome in arthritis. *Arthritis and Rheumatology* 23:137–145.

Gerdtham UG, Johannesson M (2003) A note on the effect of unemployment on mortality. *Journal of Health Economics* 22(3):505–518.

Geuskens GA, Hazes JM, Barendregt PJ, et al. (2008) Work and sick leave among patients with early inflammatory joint conditions. *Arthritis Care and Research* 59(10):1458–1466.

Gibson L, Allen S, Strong J (2002) Chapter 14. Re-integration into work. In: Strong J, Unruh AM, Wright A, Baxter GD (eds.) *Pain: A Textbook for Therapists*. London: Churchill Livingstone.

Gignac MA, Badley EM, Lacaille D, et al. (2004) Managing arthritis and employment: Making arthritis-related work changes as a means of adaptation. *American College of Rheumatology* 51(06):909–916.

Gignac MA, Cao X, Lacaille D, et al. (2008) Arthritis-related work transitions: A prospective analysis of reported productivity losses, work changes and leaving the labour force. *Arthritis Care & Research* 59(12):1805–1813.

Gilworth G, Chamberlain A, Harvey A, et al. (2003) Development of a work instability scale for rheumatoid arthritis. *Arthritis & Rheumatism* 49(3):349–354.

Hammond A, Reeve LJ, McArthur MA (2008) Occupational therapy in musculoskeletal chronic pain management. In: *British Society for Rheumatology and IASP Musculoskeletal Pain Taskforce Guidelines for the Integrated Management of Musculoskeletal Pain Symptoms (IMMsPS)* (pp.158–166). http://www.hope-academic.org.uk/Academic/researchdevelopment/Themes/Neurosciences/Pain/Guidelines_for_the_Management_of_Musculoskeletal_Pain_FINA.pdf Accessed on 15 November 2012.

Harkess J (2010) Vocational rehabilitation – A service evaluation. *The Journal of Rheumatology Occupational Therapy* 1(25):5–10.

Heasman D, Brewer P (2008) *The UK Modified Interest Checklist*. http://www.uic.edu/depts/moho/mohorelatedrsrcs#OtherInstrumentsBasedonMOHO. Accessed on 29 December 2011.

Henriksson CM, Liedberg GM, Gerdle B (2005) Women with fibromyalgia: Work and rehabilitation. *Disability & Rehabilitation* 27(12):685–695.

Hewlett S, Ambler N, Almedia C, et al. (2011) Self-management of fatigue in rheumatoid arthritis: A randomised controlled trial of group cognitive behavioural therapy. *Annals of Rheumatic Diseases* 70:1060–1067.

Jakobsen K (2001) Employment and the reconstruction of self. A model of space for maintenance of identity by occupation. *Scandinavian Journal of Occupational Therapy* 8(1):40–48.

Joss M (2007) The importance of job analysis in occupational therapy. *British Journal of Occupational Therapy* 70(7):301–303.

Kim S, Drabinski A, Williams G, et al. (2001) The impact of early rheumatoid arthritis on productivity. *Value in Health* 4(5):69.

Lacaille D (2007) Problems faced at work due to inflammatory arthritis: New insights gained from understanding patients' perspective. *Arthritis Care & Research* 57(7):11.

Law M, Baptiste S, Carswell A, et al. (1998) *The Canadian Occupational Performance Measure* (3rd edn.). Toronto, ON: CAOT Publications ACE.

Macedo AM, Oakley SP, Panayi GS, et al. (2009) Functional and work outcomes improve in patients with rheumatoid arthritis who receive targeted, comprehensive occupational therapy. *Arthritis Care & Research* 61(11):1522–1530.

Mancuso CA, Paget SA, Charlson ME (2000) Adaptations made by rheumatoid arthritis patients to continue working: A pilot study of workplace challenges and successful adaptations. *Arthritis Care & Research* 13(2):89–99.

Mathers CD, Schofield DJ (1998) The health consequences of unemployment. *Medical Journal of Australia* 168:178–182.

McArthur MA (2002) *Unheard Stories, Unmet Needs: The Clinical and Education Implication of Perceptions of Rheumatoid Arthritis*. Ph.D. thesis. Centre for Applied Research in Education, School of Education and Professional Development, University of East Anglia, Norfolk, UK.

Melvin J, Jensen G (eds.) (1998) *Rheumatologic Rehabilitation Series. Vol. 1: Assessment and Management*. Bethesda, MD: American Occupational Therapy Association.

National Institute for Clinical Excellence (NICE) (2009) *Rheumatoid Arthritis: The Management of Rheumatoid Arthritis in Adults. Clinical Guidelines 79*. www.nice.org.uk/nicemedia/pdf/CG79NICEGuideline.pdf. Accessed 19 November 2012.

National Rheumatoid Arthritis Society (NRAS) (2007) *NRAS Annual Survey. I Want to Work.* http://www.nras.org.uk/help_for_you/publications/publication_detail.aspx?id=a0B80000008Xzn2EAC. Accessed on 10 March 2012.

Newman S, Fitzpatrick R, Revenson TA, et al. (1996) *Understanding Rheumatoid Arthritis*. London: Routledge.

Osterhaus JT, Purcaru O, Richard L (2009) Discriminant validity, responsiveness and reliability of the rheumatoid arthritis-specific Work Productivity survey (WPS-RA). *Arthritis Care & Research* 11(3). http://arthritis-research.com/content/11/3/R73. Accessed on 14 November 2012.

Persson D, Andersson I, Eklund M (2011) Defying aches and re-evaluating daily doing: Occupational perspectives on adjusting to chronic pain. *Scandinavian Journal of Occupational Therapy* 18:188–197.

Puolakka K, Kautiainen H, Mottonen T, et al. (2004) Impact of initial aggressive drug treatment with a combination of disease-modifying anti-rheumatic drugs on the development of work disability in early rheumatoid arthritis: A five year randomised follow-up trial. *Arthritis and Rheumatism* 50(1):55–62.

Roessler R, Reed C, Brown P (1998) Coping with chronic illness at work: Case studies of five successful employees. *Journal of Vocational Rehabilitation* 10(3):261–269.

Ross J (2008) *Occupational Therapy and Vocational Rehabilitation*. Chichester, UK: John Wiley & Sons Ltd.

Shaw KL, Hackett J, Southwood TR, et al. (2006) The prevocational and early employment needs of adolescents with juvenile idiopathic arthritis: The adolescent perspective. *British Journal of Occupational Therapy* 69(3):98–105.

Sokka T, Kautiainen H, Pincus T, et al. (2010) Work disability remains a major problem in rheumatoid arthritis in the 2000s: Data from 32 countries in the QUEST-RA Study. *Arthritis Research & Therapy* 12:42. Open Access http://arthritis-research.com/content/pdf/ar2951.pdf. Accessed on 2 April 2012.

Stamm TA, Wright J, Machold K, et al. (2004) Occupational balance of women with rheumatoid arthritis: A qualitative study. *Musculoskeletal Care* 2(2):101–112.

Stamm TA, Machold KP, Smolen J, et al. (2010) Life Stories of people with rheumatoid arthritis who retired early: How gender and other contextual factors shaped their everyday activities, including paid work. *Musculoskeletal Care* 8(2):78–86.

Steutjens EE, Dejjer JJ, Bouter L, et al. (2008) *Occupational Therapy for Rheumatoid Arthritis* (Review). Chichester, UK: The Cochrane Collaboration. www.thecochranelibrary.com. Accessed on 14 November 2012.

Straughair S, Fawcitt S (1992) *The Road Towards Independence: The Experiences of Young People with Arthritis*. London, UK: Arthritis Care.

Varekamp I, Haafkens JA, Detaille SI, et al. (2005) Preventing work disability among employees with rheumatoid arthritis: What medical professionals can learn from the patients' perspective. *Arthritis Care & Research* 53(6):965–972.

Waddell G, Burton K (2006) *Is Work Good for Your Health and Wellbeing?* London: The Stationary Office.

Westhoff G, Buttgereit F, Gromnica-Ihle E, et al. (2008) Morning stiffness and its influence on early retirement in patients with recent onset rheumatoid arthritis. *Rheumatology* 47: 980–984.

Yelin E, Meenan R, Nevitt M, et al. (1980) Work disability in rheumatoid arthritis: Effects of disease, society, and work factors. *Annals of Internal Medicine* 93(4):551–556.

Yelin E, Henke CJ, Epstein W (1987) The work dynamics of the person with rheumatoid arthritis. *Arthritis & Rheumatism* 30(5):507–512.

Yeung R (2010) *The Extra One Per Cent: How Small Changes Make Exceptional People*. London: Pan Macmillan.

Young A, Dixey J, Kulinskaya E, et al. (2002) Which patients stop working because of rheumatoid arthritis? Results of five years' follow up in 732 patients from the Early RA Study (ERAS). *Annals of Rheumatic Diseases* 61:335–340.

Zirkzee EJM, Sneep AC, de Buck, et al. (2008) Sick leave and work disability in patients with early arthritis. *Clinical Rheumatology* 27(1):11–19.

Chapter 12

Rheumatology splinting

Sarah Bradley[1] and Jo Adams[2]

[1]*Poole Hospital NHS Foundation Trust, Dorset, United Kingdom;* [2]*University of Southampton, Southampton, United Kingdom*

12.1   Introduction

There are various important wrist and hand structures that may be affected by the inflammatory and degenerative process experienced by people with rheumatic conditions. Therefore, hand splints are a recommended conservative option for occupational therapists to prescribe to support vulnerable structures, reduce pain and optimise function and have been used for many years (Scottish Intercollegiate Guidelines Network 2002). Evidence continues to emerge regarding the clinical effectiveness of splints with the most robust evidence reporting their ability to reduce levels of wrist and hand pain when worn (Adams 2011).

This chapter introduces examples of possible splinting options for people with rheumatic conditions affecting their wrist and hands. The clinical rationale behind splint prescription is explored and the clinical decision-making process involved in splint prescription and review is considered alongside the challenges involved in measuring the outcome of rheumatological splinting.

12.2   Splinting rationale

Despite limited evidence regarding the efficacy of splinting the European League Against Rheumatism recommend splinting as a treatment that should be considered in clients with osteoarthritis (OA) affecting the hand (Zhang et al. 2007).

The beauty of splinting lies in its versatility; rather than prescribing a particular splint for a particular purpose, one splint may perform several functions. A readily available commercial splint, a wrist brace, used in many therapy departments is used to illustrate this point (Figure 12.1).

Rheumatology Practice in Occupational Therapy: Promoting Lifestyle Management, First Edition.
Edited by Lynne Goodacre and Margaret McArthur.
© 2013 John Wiley & Sons, Ltd. Published 2013 by John Wiley & Sons, Ltd.

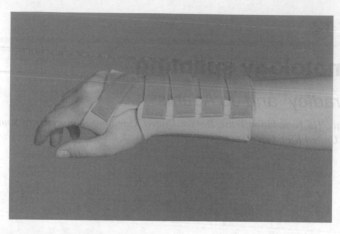

Figure 12.1   An example of a wrist brace.

Pain management

Pain affecting the hand is a feature of many rheumatological conditions and most commonly arises from primary inflammation (i.e. rheumatoid arthritis (RA)) or secondary inflammation (i.e. OA) or due to mechanical pain caused by inadequate ligamentous support, bone-on-bone contact or osteophytes impinging on soft tissues. In clinical practice, clients with RA and OA commonly report immediate relief of wrist pain on application of a wrist brace. The sustainability of pain relief on removing splints is less evident, suggesting that the effects are mainly mechanical. These anecdotal conclusions are borne out in a Cochrane review (Egan et al. 2010), which reported immediate reduction in wrist pain after donning a wrist brace. There is otherwise little evidence to support splinting for this purpose. In the absence of evidence, one can also call upon physiological knowledge to justify splinting. It is known that rest can reduce inflammation (Akeson et al. 1987), and therefore a swollen, hot rheumatoid wrist may benefit from the short-term use of a splint to assist with rapid inflammatory reduction, thus limiting joint damage.

Function

Good hand function is fundamentally important to independence; wrist braces are used to reduce functional limitation resulting from pain, weakness or wrist instability. Stern et al (1996) found that grip strength was reduced when using commercial orthoses, but this finding should be offset against the effect on wrist stability which appears to improve functional performance. A Cochrane review (Steultjens et al. 2008) drew similar conclusions regarding the use of wrist braces in the rheumatoid population, recommending that as elastic supports are inexpensive and do not appear to have any detrimental effects on range of movement (ROM) or power, they should be considered in the treatment of functional limitation until further data become available.

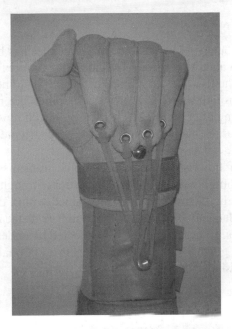

Figure 12.2   Wrist brace used with a flexion glove (Promedics).

Careful assessment grounded in sound anatomical knowledge is the foundation for understanding the pathomechanics of a dysfunctional wrist and informing the most appropriate treatment. In the absence of research evidence, biomechanical and anatomical knowledge provides a justification for splinting, e.g. an unstable distal radio-ulnar joint (DRUJ) will cause pain on loading; therefore, stabilising the DRUJ with a splint may reduce unwanted motion between the radius and ulna that reproduces pain and disrupts function.

Similarly, the wrist brace can be used to facilitate the biomechanics of other splints, e.g. in the presence of proximal inter-phalangeal joint (PIPJ) contractures, a wrist brace may be used beneath a flexion glove to prevent unwanted and compensatory flexion through the wrist, allowing the flexion glove to act upon the PIPJs. Using a splint in this manner is described as a torque transmission splint (Fess et al. 2005) as it allows motion to be inhibited in one area to facilitate movement in another. There is conflicting evidence as to the efficacy of mobilisation splinting in the rheumatoid population; however, a gentle, slow, sustained pull applied to un-inflamed tissues can lead to improvement in soft tissue contracture (Brand 2002).

The wrist brace shown in Figure 12.2 is used with a flexion glove (Promedics), to increase passive range of motion in the digits. A screw rivet has been attached to the splint at the proximal end as the attachment for the elastic bands. This has the advantage on increasing the leverage of the elastic bands to produce greater force if desired. It also prevents flexion of the wrist allowing the forces of motion to be directed specifically to the fingers.

Joint protection

The significant contribution of joint protection principles has been recognised in the NICE guidance on RA and OA (National Collaborating Centre for Chronic Conditions 2008; NICE 2009). The use of a wrist brace can facilitate joint protection principles by reducing stress through the carpus or DRUJ. Splints are recommended for this purpose in the 'Looking after your joints leaflet' produced by Arthritis Research UK (ARUK 2012) and can be helpful when aiming to distribute loads when carrying heavy objects.

One must consider however the effects of force transmission to unconstrained joints, e.g. if using a thumb/wrist splint to reduce stress through the base of the thumb some force will be redirected to joints unconstrained within the splint during function, i.e. the inter-phalangeal joint (IPJ) of the thumb or metacarpal phalangeal joints (MCPJs) of the fingers. If these joints are also affected by underlying pathology, then consideration must be given to educating the client in additional joint protection strategies such as using assistive devices.

Post surgery

Wrist braces can be useful following surgical procedures affecting the wrist. Arthrodesis is a reliable procedure undertaken in both the OA and RA wrist; the rehabilitation phase of treatment can be an anxious time for clients who are unsure how much loading their fused wrist can take. A soft step down splint can ease the client's transition to confident function following removal of a cast.

A wrist brace may also be used as a torque transmission splint. Following MCPJ arthroplasty, e.g., clients may struggle to flex their new joints due to pre-operative weakness, and in trying to regain movement have compensatory movement at the wrist rather than the MCPs because joints with less resistance and greater power move more readily. A wrist brace can be used during exercise to inhibit wrist motion and therefore direct motion to the MCPs where it is required.

The wrist brace is an example of a cheap and readily available commercial orthosis and has been used to demonstrate the ability of a splint to achieve several different therapeutic goals. There is a large commercial market for the wrist brace; with budgetary constraints being a significant consideration in the selection of orthoses therapists need to consider that not all wrist braces are the same. The properties of different materials, e.g. neoprene and elastic and different designs, may impact on the specific goal of splinting.

The occupational therapist is therefore required to employ a combination of evidence and clinical reasoning skills to inform the clinical decision-making process, with the client at the centre. The research findings cited in this section should be interpreted and applied with caution as most studies predate the more aggressive medical management of RA in particular. The future presentation and problems facing the person with RA may present different challenges. There is still much to be explored and understood about splinting as a treatment modality. Until more robust evidence exists, therapists should focus in clinical practice on measuring the effectiveness of splinting interventions to ensure that the aims of splinting are achieved on an individual basis to justify its continued use.

12.3 Clinical decision making

The decision to splint a person with a rheumatic condition can be challenging and should be driven by their individual needs identified through an accurate process of assessment. Before embarking upon splinting, the therapist should have a clear understanding of the pathology, pathomechanics and biologic state of the tissues involved as well as an appreciation of the uniqueness of the individual's needs. Splint design, materials used and prescription for use will ultimately depend on the purpose and function of the splint which include:

- supporting and resting weakened structures,
- improving joint positioning,
- minimising contractures and
- improving function (Fess et al. 2005)

The importance of the client's goals and needs have been highlighted earlier; however, the clinical reasoning for splinting has many layers and can be complex. To demonstrate, these 'layers' have been separated into three categories:

- Disease management
- client management
- Management of mechanical function/dysfunction

Each of these categories will be discussed and an example of how splinting contributes to each is provided.

Disease management

In all the inflammatory arthropathies, swelling and synovitis are common features of the disease. Unmanaged inflammation can cause damage to joints and soft tissue, which can lead to mechanical derangement, deformities and impaired function (Falconer 1991). Despite significant improvements in medical management, inflammation still occurs to a destructive level in many clients (Mamehara et al. 2010). This can be identified through clinical observation and assessment, tender joint counts and reviewing the client's most recent blood tests which may indicate raised erythrosedimentation rate and/or C-reactive protein. In OA, inflammation may be secondary and significantly limit function due to pain. Providing the client with tools to manage inflammation such as splints which temporarily rest the painful swollen joints may therefore be helpful.

For many years, resting splints were used alongside advice to rest and immobilise wrist and hand joints. However, management of RA has changed; drug regimes are

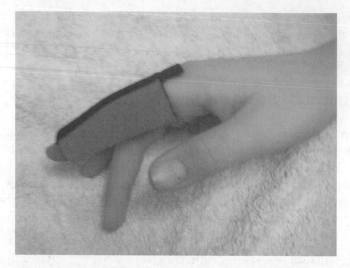

Figure 12.3   A circumferential sleeve made with neoprene or Comfortprene (Promedics). The tape ironed on the dorsal surface secures the seam which avoids the need to sew it. It also creates an extension force; the resting posture of the index finger is much straighter than the adjacent digits. Additionally, the tape is folded in a flap at the proximal end to allow for easier donning/doffing.

now more effective, and inflammation is often controlled much more effectively. Recent research undertaken with people with RA in the early stages of the disease (less than 5 years) suggests that using resting splints to immobilise wrist and hand joints alongside more effective drug regimes may lead to limited improvements in clients' functional movements (Adams 2008). However, alongside this study, Silva et al. (2008) conducted a randomised controlled trial recruiting clients with longer standing RA (average 10 years) who reported significant improvement in pain levels over 90 days as a result of wearing resting splints.

There is otherwise little contemporary evidence around splinting effects in disease management. Despite this immobilisation, splinting in other forms remains a popular choice in therapy departments for disease management. Short-term immobilisation splinting can take many forms; there are various thermoplastic designs, customised neoprene splints and off-the-shelf options. The choice of splint will depend on the client's presentation, the skills of the therapist in terms of splint construction and the resources available.

As a case example, swelling and pain affecting the PIPJ is very common in many types of rheumatological disease. The neoprene sleeve (Figure 12.3) is a valuable treatment in this scenario; its circumferential and elastic properties allow it to both splint and provide compression to reduce swelling, which in turn reduces pain and improves motion.

It is cheap to make, can be applied to multiple digits and as the client's pain resolves, allows some movement whilst maintaining compression. On its own, it is strong enough to provide stability to an unstable PIPJ. Neoprene sleeves can also be

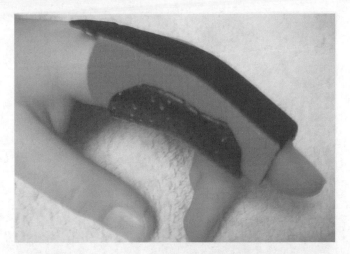

Figure 12.4   The neoprene sleeve can be reinforced on the volar surface with thermoplastic to prevent flexion at the PIPJ, e.g. where active extension is compromised by a boutonniere deformity.

used in conjunction with thermoplastic, e.g. if strict immobilisation is required to manage an acute boutonniere deformity, it can be reinforced volarly with materials such as Orfit© to prevent PIPJ flexion but still allow distal interphalangeal (DIP) movement (Figure 12.4). Whatever the choice of design, short-term immobilisation is preferable to long-term immobilisation due to the risks associated with tissue health (Akeson et al. 1987).

Management of the client

Therapists will always encounter clients whose circumstances do not allow the 'ideal' treatment to be offered. The elderly population are one such example as new biologic therapies were not available at the onset of their disease, meaning they will have to live with the deformities and instabilities which occurred in the early stages of their disease. Whilst surgery may be a solution to joint pain and poor function in this group of clients, coexisting problems may preclude this option due to general health risks, poor bone stock and poor skin condition leading to healing risks; assessment of cognitive ability may highlight an inability to cope with post-operative therapy. We still however have a duty of care to provide such clients with a treatment that is right for them. In this scenario, careful examination of the client's priorities is paramount in addressing their needs.

Splints may form part of the treatment programme if the problem is pain, weakness and instability, or correctable deformity. Whilst it is accepted that wearing an immobilisation splint permanently is detrimental to joint health, where significant joint destruction has already occurred and is irreparable, this may be the only solution to managing pain during function. Furthermore, some clients opt out of surgery,

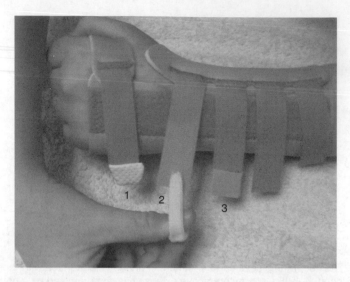

Figure 12.5   A wrist brace showing examples of adapted straps: (1) Thermoplastic is used to reinforce the end of the strap leaving it free to grasp; (2) a strip of strapping was used to create a loop – this is held open with a small thermoplastic strip for easy finger insertion and (3) a strip of tape used to seal seams on neoprene was ironed on to create a tab.

e.g. following attrition ruptures of extensor pollicis longus in favour of splinting to maintain function. Therapists may have witnessed in this client group their proficient ability to adapt and compensate for their impairment. This only increases the challenge for splints to improve hand function and highlights the importance of measuring outcomes following splinting.

Another factor influencing splint choice is the ability of the client to apply it. This is a particular challenge in this group of clients due to the bilateralism of RA. Occupational therapists must be vigilant in such matters or the splint will not be worn and therapeutic goals not achieved. Creativity is essential to adapting splints to facilitate uptake of the wearing schedule (Figure 12.5).

Managing the client and their expectations is complex; therefore, clear documentation of the client's goals/needs and the clinical reasoning surrounding and justifying the therapist's treatment prescription are essential. Like all treatments, comprehensive, written advice should be given to clients so that they are clear about the expectations for the splint and what is required of them to achieve their goals.

Management of mechanical dysfunction

Hand and wrist deformity occurs in people with rheumatic conditions in many forms, including MCPJ ulnar deviation due to capsular attenuation and joint destruction, PIPJ flexion contractures due to skin contractures in scleroderma, or subluxation of the metacarpal on the trapezium as commonly seen in OA affecting the carpometacarpal joint (CMCJ). Early identification of deformity through a thorough and detailed assessment of biomechanical dysfunction can be very successfully managed with splinting (Biese 2002). As a case example, one of the most disabling and common deformities affecting the hand is the swan neck deformity characterised by hyper-extension of the PIPJ and flexion at the DIP. The pathomechanics of this deformity are complex and can arise from the MCP, PIP or DIP, thereby demonstrating how important careful assessment is to ensure the most appropriate and effective splint is applied.

MCP joint

Proliferative synovitis at the MCPJs leads to volar subluxation and ulnar devia-tion. As this occurs, the resting tension of the intrinsic muscles relaxes and the muscles shorten; this action of the intrinsic tendon increases the extension force on the PIPJ, thus hyperextending it (Alter et al. 2002). Deformity at this level can be assessed using Bunnell's test of intrinsic tightness (Welsh and Hastings 1977). As the deformity progresses and as the MCPJ is extended the potential for PIPJ flexion decreases; conversely, when the MCP is flexed, PIPJ is allowed further flexion.

In this scenario, treatment needs to be directed at treating the intrinsic tightness. To do this exercise, splints or torque transmission splinting is most useful. A volar-based splint should be applied to the hand that supports the MCPJs in maximal extension; care must be taken to ensure there is no hyperextension at the MCP but that the joint is fully supported in neutral. The fingers are then left free from the PIPJ and regular cycles of flexion/extension performed to maximally achievable flexion. Over several weeks/months, the intrinsic muscles should lengthen again. Intermittent splinting is likely to be required to maintain the tendon balance achieved. In cases of extreme intrinsic tightness, dynamic or static progressive splinting may be necessary to exert greater passive forces on the shortened muscles (Prosser and Conolly 2003).

PIP joint

Synovitis stretches out the volar capsule and plate which allows the PIPJ to hyperextend. The lateral bands then migrate dorsally, relaxing tension on the terminal extensor and causing the DIP to rest in flexion. In severe cases, the flexor digitorum superficialis tendon can rupture, which further fixes the deformity (Alter et al. 2002).

In this scenario, splinting at the PIPJ level to correct hyperextension would be helpful. Bringing the PIPJ into flexion will help to restore tendon imbalance and bring the digit into a more functional position for grasp. This can be achieved through dorsally blocking the PIP with a ring splint. These can be purchased from orthotics suppliers in the form of oval-8 splints or bespoke silver rings such as those reported by Spicka et al. (2009). The deformity at this level is often permanent and therefore splinting is a long-term requirement, so the splint selected needs to be tolerable for long periods. A graded wearing schedule is often useful to ensure skin integrity is

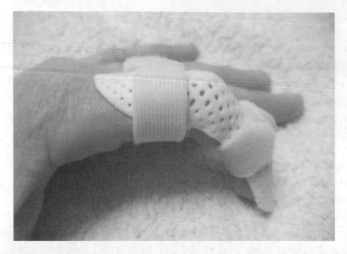

Figure 12.6   A dorsal blocking splint made in a 1.6mm material is moulded on the dorsal surface to maintain flexion at the PIPJ at night to facilitate correction of swan neck deformity.

maintained. A dorsally based gutter splint moulded into flexion is useful to maintain desirable PIPJ flexion at night (Figure 12.6).

DIP joint

At the DIP, synovitis can lead to attenuation or rupture of the terminal extensor tendon, which leads to a mallet deformity (Alter et al. 2002). Extensor force is therefore directed more proximally to the PIPJ causing hyperextension, especially when associated with an already lax volar plate.

A mallet-type splint that restores DIP extension is the treatment of choice. These are available as prefabricated splints commonly used in accident and emergency departments, or can be custom made to fit either dorsally or volarly. It is critical however that the PIPJ is free and allowed to flex fully to prevent unwanted stiffness (Anderson 2011).

In all cases, there are no rules regarding wearing schedule, therapists should determine this based on the biologic state of the tissues involved, the severity of the deformity and the practical implications imposed by the splint within the context of the client's life.

Despite the origins of the deformity, splinting can only be effective if the deformity is passively correctable (Porter and Brittain 2012). Therapists should also consider that splints may improve mechanical components but impair sensory components of function; functional usefulness must therefore be evaluated on an individual level.

Splinting is most likely to be effective when combined with medical management, joint protection, strengthening and pain reduction techniques; therefore, future research evaluation should probably occur within the context of these other treatments.

12.4   Approaches to evaluation

The approach to evaluating the effectiveness of a splint will relate to the aims of splinting. The earlier sections of this chapter have highlighted the importance of a client-centred splint regime to target and to improve the possible impairments associated with rheumatological conditions. These may include joint synovitis and pain, reduced range of joint movement and reduced muscle strength. Occupational therapists are particularly concerned with how the impact of these impairments may affect hand and overall function such as the impact on dexterity, grip strength and hand co-ordination and the influence these may have on the ability to participate in valued daily activities. Thus, in order to evaluate the effectiveness of splints, the outcome measures chosen need to capture the key level(s) of functioning which the splint intervention aims to target. The measures also need to reflect those issues which are important to the client and others as different individuals may have different priorities. For example, a carer may be most concerned that their partner has sufficient wrist flexion to independently carry out their personal hygiene tasks, the occupational therapist may be focusing on the ROM of the wrist to ensure that the wrist and hand biomechanics are addressed to allow this functional movement thus fore, different outcome measures may be required to capture these different priorities.

The outcome measures used to evaluate splint and hand therapy require careful consideration. Not only do they need to demonstrate robust psychometric properties (ideally reported within the same diagnostic group of clients), but they also need to provide useful information that is easy to score and report and is relevant for both client and therapist. So, measures need to have evidence that they are valid, reliable and responsive to clinically meaningful change (Bowling 2000) and therapists need to be conversant with how responsive an outcome may be to the aim of the splinting intervention. Published evidence will guide a decision as to the most useful outcome measure to use when measuring different impairment, functional and participation domains.

Evaluation of the effectiveness of splints should consist of client-reported outcome measures (PROMs), standardised therapist assessed outcomes and clinical review. Examples of PROMs include:

- A 100 mm pain or hand function Visual Analogue Scale
- The Quick Disability of the Arm, Shoulder and Hand (DASH) questionnaire (Beaton et al. 2005)
- The Michigan Hand Questionnaire (Chung et al. 1998)
- The AUSCAN Osteoarthritis Hand Index (Bellamy et al. 2002)

Examples of appropriate therapist-assessed measures include functional hand tests that capture global hand function such as:

- The Grip Ability Test (GAT) (Dellhag and Bjelle 1995)
- The Arthritis Hand Function Test (Backman et al. 1990)

Clinical review will be based upon the occupational therapist and wider team evaluating the progress of the disease and any resulting impairments and functional limitations and reviewing the continued impact of the splint. If the disease and hand functional ability have changed, then the splint needs to be adjusted accordingly.

All of the standardised measures mentioned earlier have evidence of sound psychometric properties in evaluating hand and upper limb outcome in people with rheumatic conditions. Each outcome measure will have different positive features. Some provide benchmark reference values for classifying functional status (Backman et al. 1990); others perform particularly well in registering change in this population (Chung et al. 1998); and others such as the GAT (Dellhag and Bjelle 1995) are inexpensive to construct and easy to use in a department. Some measures are quick to conduct and score such as the Joint Alignment and Motion Scale (Spiegel et al. 1987); others such as the Canadian Occupational Performance Measure (Law et al. 1990) are particularly well suited to recording the client's own goals and objectives for treatment and may also be a useful tool, particularly so that clients can identify their key issues for improvement.

No one outcome measure will be perfect, and the skill lies in identifying one that is relevant for the client and therapist and will register clinically important change over the intervention time. The latter point is becoming increasingly important for departments defending and justifying splinting budgets.

Issues to consider when evaluating splints

There is however little compelling evidence for splinting, which may be due to the multifaceted nature of splinting and musculoskeletal disease adding complexity to evaluation.

Occupational therapists need to not only consider how they review splints and with which outcome measures but also the timing of the review; thinking carefully about whether the splint has been worn for sufficient time to effect a change, i.e. is the splint 'dosage' sufficient to have had an effect? This relates to whether clients have been provided with a standardised wearing regime or advised to wear their splints 'as and when' they feel necessary.

Strategies to enhance exercise concordance using cognitive behavioural approaches have already been implemented within RA populations with good effect (Heine et al. 2012), and these can easily be applied to splint wear regimes too, e.g. the use of intention diaries where individuals document when and for how long they will wear their splint making a written record of their behaviour. A positive approach from all team members regarding the effectiveness of splinting can also play its part in encouraging the client to develop higher levels of outcome expectancy and in turn encourage splint wear adherence (Feinberg 1992; Groth and Wulf 1995).

One challenging issue for therapists when recording the effectiveness of splints is that there are many factors that may impact upon measurable functional outcome, e.g. disease process. A person's underlying condition may be progressive or characterised by acute flare or remission; thus it could be that any improvement made by the splint intervention is obscured by a disease flare or progression. Therefore, disease status needs to be taken into account when recording splint outcome so that the interpretation of outcome is adjusted accordingly.

The provision of splints for people with rheumatic conditions will usually be only part of the intervention programme provided by the occupational therapist and team members. Splints may be provided alongside exercise, joint protection, fatigue management and pain management strategies. As such, they serve as only one part of a complex package of care. Trying to work out accurately the part that splints contribute to this overall package is difficult without the evidence of qualitative and quantitative research studies. Evaluating and attributing splinting outcome is therefore important but complex.

12.5   Splint construction

Splints may be commercially made 'off-the-shelf' options or custom made by therapists. Here, we introduce examples of six splints that may be used in rheumatology, highlighting the potential strengths of each design.

Off-the-shelf splints

Elastic wrist based support

This splint has been used for many years and has been seen to reduce hand pain (Pagnotta et al. 2005). It is important that off-the-shelf options are made to fit the individual. This will involve adjusting any supportive palmar inserts or bars integral to the splint and ensuring that fastenings are accessible and practical for the client.

Thumb posts (Colditz Push splint)

This is an exciting new splint that has generated much interest amongst clients and therapists. The splint works by immobilising the first metacarpal but allowing all other joints to move freely. It is particularly useful in early OA where MCP hyperextension has not developed and allows MCP flexion which is known to offload the CMCJ during function. Client feedback is positive about this splint, and during service user involvement groups for a thumb base trial people have reported that it is easy to fasten, is lightweight and is comfortable (Gooberman-Hill et al. 2012).

Oval 8's PIPJ

These are simple thermoplastic three-point splints that apply pressure across the proximal and middle phalanges and passively correct deformity at the distal interphalangeal joint (DIPJ) or PIPJ. They can help to prevent and control swan necking of the PIPJ, lateral deviation of the hand joints and boutonniere deformity. PIP and DIP anatomy is so intimately interconnected that disease at one joint will affect motion at the other. Deformity at these joints has significant implications for people's function and dexterity (Adams 2008).

Custom-made splints

Exercise splints

Exercise splints take many forms but are usually made of thermoplastic material. Using anatomical knowledge, the splint can be used to facilitate the direction of motion to the joint/tissues being exercised by inhibiting motion that interferes with this motion being achieved, e.g. in the case of intrinsic tightness, MCPs are splinted in extension where intrinsics are under greater tension; the PIPs are free in the splint and are flexed to stretch the intrinsics further. Repeated cycles of exercise over time will lead to lengthening of the intrinsic muscles. A small, simple gutter fabricated in a scrap of material such as Orfilight or tailorsplint can be fitted over the IPJ of the thumb to facilitate flexor pollicis brevis action following thumb MCPJ arthroplasty.

Neoprene sleeves

Neoprene is an extremely versatile material that is available in different thicknesses and many colours making it suitable for all age groups. They are very simple and cheap to make with limited training and can be machine washed. An example of their application is described in the section on disease management. It has also been used to give support to PIPJs, destroyed by mutilans disease, that are very unstable and consequently painful. The sleeve provides support and prevents repeated dislocation that occurs when functioning.

Silver splints

Most recently, therapists have been involved in developing custom-made splints using different approaches and materials. In the UK, Christina Macleod has worked collaboratively with a high-street jeweller to create beautiful but functional, hard-wearing bespoke silver splints that clients enjoy wearing (Macleod and Adams 2002). This innovative and novel approach to providing small finger-based splints and one off splints typifies the creative approach of an occupational therapist to produce effective client-centred solutions.

People who use these splints report that they are pleased to wear something that does not look like a medical orthotic and are delighted with how attractive they are. The issue of body image is always important when considering hand splinting:

> I wouldn't be hiding my hands with these…but with the plastic ones I was trying to hide them behind my back.…'With these I don't feel so ashamed.'

> Because they make you feel good, wearing them you're not so conscious about the deformity and they just make you feel better which is a good thing. I think when you got RA, you're so conscious of all the deformities you know the pain and the ugly joints and things - they make you feel like a proper woman. (Spicka et al. 2008).

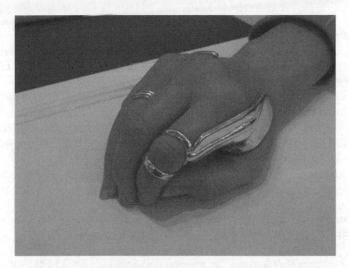

Figure 12.7 Example of a functional hand-based orthosis.

Having the scope to be creative in splint making can bring real rewards. The splint illustrated in Figure 12.7 was tailor made for a woman with RA who wanted to continue to horse ride at a competitive level. The splint supports her index finger sufficiently to exert the amount of pressure and force required to hold, feel and respond to the reins in her hand. Without the additional support, this woman was unable to control her horse in the required way.

12.6 Summary

So in sum, this chapter has introduced some commonly used splints and considered some more recent splinting options. The client-centred approach to splinting has indicated that a problem-based approach to splinting should be encouraged. The underlying disease process and the possible associated hand impairment and functional limitations will guide the occupational therapist's management approach. One splint may be used for different purposes, and there is scope for creativity in design. The evidence for the effectiveness of splinting is still being established. Choosing the appropriate tools to evaluate the usefulness of splints will continue to help establish which splints benefit which people at what time.

References

Adams J (2008) Three dimensional functional motion analysis of silver ring splints in rheumatoid arthritis. *Rheumatology* 47(Suppl 2):ii154.

Adams J (2011) Orthotics of the hand. In: Dziedzic K, Hammond A (eds.) *Rheumatology: Evidence Based Practice for Physiotherapists and Occupational Therapists* (pp. 163–170). Edinburgh, UK: Elsevier.

Akeson WH, Amiel D, Abel MF, et al. (1987) Effects of immobilization on joints. *Clinical Orthopaedics and Related Research* 219:28–37.

Alter S, Feldon P, Torrono AL (2002) Pathomechanics of deformities in the arthritic hand and wrist. In: Hunter JM, Laverty J, Pollock R, et al. (eds.) *Rehabilitation of the Hand and Upper Extremity* (5th edn.). St Louis, MO: Mosby.

Anderson D (2011) Mallet finger: Management and patient compliance. *Australian Family Physician* 40:47–48.

Arthritis Research UK (ARUK) (2012) *Looking After Your Joints.* http://www.arthritisresearchuk. org/~/media/Files/Arthritis-information/Living-with-arthritis/2055-Looking-after-your-joints. ashx. Accessed on 14 November 2012.

Backman C, Mackie H, Harris J (1990) Arthritis hand function test: Development of a standardised assessment tool. In: *Canadian Association of Occupational Therapists Conference 1990.* Toronto, ON: CAOT Publications.

Beaton D, Wright J, Katz J, Upper Extremity Group (2005) Development of the QuickDASH: Comparison of three item-reduction approaches. *Journal of Bone Joint Surgery* 87:1038–1046.

Bellamy N, Campbell J, Haraoui B, et al. (2002) Dimensionality and clinical importance of pain and disability in hand osteoarthritis: Development of the Australian/Canadian (AUSCAN) Osteoarthritis Hand Index. *Osteoarthritis Cartilage* 10(11):855–862.

Biese J (2002) Therapists evaluation and conservative management of rheumatoid arthritis in the hand and wrist. In: Hunter JM, Laverty J, Pollock R, et al. (eds.) *Rehabilitation of the Hand and Upper Extremity* (5th edn.). St Louis, MO: Mosby.

Bowling A (2000) *Measuring Disease* (2nd edn.). Buckingham, UK: Open University Press.

Brand P (2002) Lessons from hot feet: A note on tissue remodelling. *Journal of Hand Therapy* 15(2):133–135.

Chung KC, Pillsbury MS, Walters MR, et al. (1998) Reliability and validity testing of the Michigan Hand Outcomes Questionnaire. *The Journal of Hand Surgery* 23A(4): 575–587.

Dellhag B, Bjelle A (1995) A grip ability test for use in rheumatology practice. *The Journal of Rheumatology* 22(8):1559–1565.

Egan E, Brosseau L, Farmer M, et al. (2010) Splints and orthoses for treating rheumatoid arthritis. *Cochrane Database of Systematic Reviews* 4: Art. no.: CD004018.

Falconer J (1991) Hand splinting in Rheumatoid arthritis. A perspective on current knowledge and directions for research. *Arthritis Care and Research* 4(2):81–85.

Feinberg J (1992) The effect of the arthritis health care professional on compliance with the use of resting hand splints by patients with rheumatoid arthritis. *Arthritis Care and Research* 5(1):17–23.

Fess EE, Gettle KS, Philips CA (2005) *Hand and Upper Extremity Splinting. Principles and Methods* (3rd edn.). St Louis, MO: Elsevier Mosby.

Gooberman-Hill R, Jinks C, Barbosa Bouças S, et al. (2012) Involving service users in trial design outcomes, splint selection and placebo design in a trial of treatment for thumb-base osteoarthritis. *Rheumatology* 51(Suppl 3):54–55.

Groth GN, Wulf MB (1995) Compliance with hand rehabilitation: Health beliefs and strategies. *Journal of Hand Therapy* 8(1):18–22.

Heine PJ, Williams MA, Williamson E, et al. (2012) Development and delivery of an exercise intervention for rheumatoid arthritis: Strengthening and stretching for rheumatoid arthritis of the hand (SARAH) trial. *Physiotherapy* 98(2):121–130.

Law M, Baptiste S, McColl M, et al. (1990) The Canadian occupational performance measure: An outcome measure for occupational therapy. *Canadian Journal of Occupational Therapy* 57(2):82–87.

Macleod C, Adams J (2002) Improving patient adherence to swan neck ring splints. *Rheumatology* 41(Suppl 1):89.

Mamehara A, Sugimoto T, Sugiyama D, et al. (2010) 1, Serum Matrix Metalloproteinase-3 as predictor of joint destruction in rheumatoid arthritis, treated with non-biological disease modifying anti-rheumatic drugs Kobe. *Journal of Medical Sciences* 56(3): E98–E107.

National Collaborating Centre for Chronic Conditions (2008) *Osteoarthritis: National Clinical Guideline for Care and Management in Adults.* London: Royal College of Physicians.

National Institute for Health and Clinical Excellence (NICE) (2009) *Rheumatoid Arthritis. National Clinical Guideline for Management and Treatment in Adults.* NICE Clinical Guideline 79.

Pagnotta A, Korner-Bitensky N, Mazer B, et al. (2005) Static wrist splint use in the performance of daily activities by individuals with rheumatoid arthritis. *Journal of Rheumatology* 32(11):2136–2143.

Porter BJ, Brittain A (2012) Splinting and hand exercise for three common hand deformities in rheumatoid arthritis: A clinical perspective. *Current Opinion in Rheumatology* 24(2):215–221.

Prosser R, Conolly WB (2003) Rheumatoid arthritis. In: Prosser R, Conolly WB (eds.) *Rehabilitation of the Hand and Upper Limb.* Edinburgh, UK: Butterworth Heineman.

Scottish Intercollegiate Guidelines Network (2002) *Management of Early Arthritis.* Section 5 The Role of the multidisciplinary team. http://www.sign.ac.uk/pdf/sign123.pdf. Accessed on 21 November 2012.

Silva AC, Jones A, Silva PG, et al. (2008) Effectiveness of a night-time hand positioning splint in rheumatoid arthritis: A randomized controlled trial. *Journal of Rehabilitation Medicine* 40(9):749–754.

Spicka C, Adams J, Macleod C, et al. (2008) A study examining the effectiveness of silver ring splints in adult patient with rheumatoid arthritis. *Rheumatology* 47(Suppl 2):ii33–ii34.

Spicka C, Adams J, Macleod C, et al. (2009) The effectiveness of silver ring splints in adult patients with rheumatoid arthritis. *Hand Therapy* 14:53–57.

Spiegel TM, Spiegel JS, Paulus HE (1987) The joint alignment and motion scale: A simple measure of joint deformity in patients with rheumatoid arthritis. *The Journal of Rheumatology* 145:887–892.

Stern EB, Ytterberg SR, Krug HE, et al. (1996) Immediate and short term effects of three commercial wrist extensor orthoses on grip strength and function in patients with rheumatoid arthritis. *Arthritis Care and Research* 9(1):42–50.

Steultjens EE, Dekker JJ, Bouter L, et al. (2008) Occupational therapy for rheumatoid arthritis. *Cochrane Database of Systematic Reviews* (1): Art. no. CD003114.

Welsh R, Hastings D (1997) Swan neck deformity in rheumatoid arthritis. *The Hand* 9(22):109–116.

Zhang W, Doherty M, Leeb BF, et al. (2007) EULAR evidence based recommendations for the management of hand osteoarthritis: Report of a task force of the EULAR Standing Committee for International Clinical Studies Including Therapeutics (ESCISIT). *Annals of Rheumatic Disease* 66:377–388.

Chapter 13

Maintaining a sense of self

Penny Sloane[1] and Lynne Goodacre[2]

[1]*Penny Sloane Associates, London, United Kingdom;* [2]*Lancaster University, Lancaster, United Kingdom*

13.1 Introduction

Self-concept is a multidimensional construct comprising a person's perception of themselves in relation to a range of characteristics such as beliefs about personal qualities, skills and abilities, social roles, body image and sexual identity. It refers in essence to how one views one's self as a person, i.e. 'who I am' (Cronin Mosley 1986). Self-esteem is an evaluative component of self-concept representing the degree to which we ascribe worth to ourselves (Cronin Mosley 1986) informed not only by our thoughts and feelings but by comparisons with others and how others react to us.

Previous chapters have outlined the significant impact of rheumatic conditions on all aspects of a person's life. In this chapter, we will develop this by focusing on body image and personal and sexual relationships areas, often neglected in the clinical management of people with rheumatic conditions. We will introduce some strategies that can be utilised to help address some of the challenges that people may experience in these aspects of their lives.

To provide the context for this chapter, Penny has written a personal narrative which conveys aspects of her experience of living with rheumatoid arthritis (RA) and her personal journey to becoming a professional image consultant (see Box 13.1).

Penny's narrative illustrates the impact of RA on many highly valued aspects of her life; such lifestyle disruptions have been described as *illness intrusions* (Devins 2006; Devins et al. 1992) which interfere with a person's continued involvement in valued activities. In studying the personal impact of RA on peoples' identity, Lempp et al. (2006) highlighted a number of areas in which identity was affected (Table 13.1).

Rheumatology Practice in Occupational Therapy: Promoting Lifestyle Management, First Edition.
Edited by Lynne Goodacre and Margaret McArthur.
© 2013 John Wiley & Sons, Ltd. Published 2013 by John Wiley & Sons, Ltd.

Box 13.1   Penny's personal narrative

Rheumatoid arthritis hit me at the age of 27 like a bolt from the blue. At the time I was living and working in London and had a very successful career as a Senior Buyer for Marks & Spencer. It started with pains in my shoulders – a type of pain I'd never experienced before, nothing I did alleviated it. It moved around my body, never settling in one place. One day I'd be unable to move my fingers, the next my elbow would lock. For some time there was no diagnosis and because I'd have good days and bad days there were periods when it seemed that no-one, not even my GP, really believed that I felt so unwell. Looking back, my overwhelming feeling was that I was frightened. The pain and debilitating nature of RA was not only a shock but also something I felt too young to be experiencing and ill-equipped to deal with.

I was diagnosed 6 months before I got married and the initial treatment kept things relatively under control. We had our first baby and the RA, which had worsened (unusually) during pregnancy, became even worse postpartum. I decided to stop working – I was exhausted and in constant pain but I went on to have another three children. I remember being advised against this but I couldn't and wouldn't allow my RA to dictate my family life. Gradually, over time I became more disabled. I used the pushchair as my walking frame and I had to use my forearms to pick my babies up as my hands were so swollen and sore.

I remember two hospital visits in particular that I found deeply depressing. The first was to visit an occupational therapist. As I sat looking at the different aids that would make my life easier I wanted to weep because it really brought home that I wasn't 'normal'. The second was to pick up some boots that had been made for me. I had such high hopes, I'd helped design them and at last I felt I'd have some footwear that might look reasonably normal and semi-attractive. I opened the box with great excitement but the boots were awful, orthopaedic monstrosities; I would rather not have walked than worn them. I went home and threw several hundred pounds worth of bespoke footwear in the bin.

On reflection, the services offered were probably the best available and meant to help me become more enabled. However, they had the opposite effect psychologically and just made me feel less normal, less a part of the ordinary world, more singled out, more different. I absolutely hated any show of pity from anyone and so developed all sorts of strategies to hide my RA and I was certainly not going to use anything that I felt would mark me out as different.

Of course, things change and there came a time when it was clear that I was facing some severe restrictions on living my life the way I had expected. I was unable to walk without sticks and, if I needed to get up in the night, I often had to crawl to the loo. I felt humiliated by my disease, I couldn't find a drug regime that worked and I continued on a downward spiral until, in 2003, I began anti-TNF therapy and underwent joint replacement surgery.

For the first time in years, the chronic, grinding pain lessened and I began to see some light at the end of the tunnel. However, by this time, my self-confidence and self- esteem had hit rock bottom and I had become unable to do things I'd always taken for granted. RA had also changed my self-perception and in many ways that was the hardest thing to deal with.

I had put on a significant amount of weight over years of taking steroids, and together with being less active, I felt frumpy and old fashioned. When I looked at my body, particularly the bits on show that had become disfigured like my hands, I felt that was all others would see. However, because I had started to feel somewhat better I decided to try and lift myself out of the mire. So, I lost weight and then decided to have a consultation with an Image Consultant. She came to my home and we spent the day looking at style, colour and the contents of my wardrobe. It was a fantastic day – literally life changing.

By the time she left, I had been able to get back in touch with aspects of the person I'd been before my life had been overtaken by RA. I suddenly felt that somehow I had been given permission to be glamorous, attractive and sexy again, all aspects of myself that I had lost touch with. I realised that I could think less about the bits of me that had gone wrong and more about making the most of the rest of me. I began to see myself in a different way, the arthritis lost some of its power and was consigned to being a part of me rather than what defined me. Such was the effect that this session had and so great was the feeling of transformation that I undertook training to become an Image Consultant.

It is very hard to think of yourself as vibrant, attractive and part of the 'normal' world when you have been devastated by an illness such as arthritis. To some degree, you lose control and the disease takes over, altering you physically in a way that is obvious to others and so marks you out. I have learned that feeling good about your appearance is very empowering and can have an enormously beneficial effect on self-esteem and mental well-being. Developing strategies that give greater self-confidence makes you feel happier and better physically, as well as mentally, because you regain a sense of power and control.

Table 13.1 Ways in which identity can be affected by rheumatic conditions.

Within the private sphere	Within the public domain
• Emotional identity – feeling 'low' • Identity as a parent/carer • Identity as an independent person • Identity as a partner	• Identity as an employee • Identity as a friend • Public identity (stigmatisation and discrimination)
Within the private and public sphere	
• Physical identity (physical appearance) • Loss of social roles • Self-image	

Studies exploring the impact of rheumatic conditions on the performance of valued life activities have identified consistently the link between reduced ability to engage in valued life activities and psychological well-being (Katz et al. 2006; Reinseth and Espnes 2007; Reinseth et al. 2010). It is important to emphasise that what is highly valued by one person may not be by another (Katz and Yelin 2001), reinforcing the need for a person-centred approach to working which focuses on the priorities and values of clients (Devins 2006).

13.2 Impact of rheumatic conditions on body experience

Living in and with a body which is changing is a universal experience. Our bodies develop along an expected trajectory, and we have a good idea about what this means in terms of our changing appearance. We have differing views about how much time and money we are willing to invest in trying to arrest such change and place differing values on the importance of the image we portray and the way we present ourselves.

Concerns about appearance in Western societies have been described as reaching epidemic proportions (Rumsey and Harcourt 2005, p. 63) and dissatisfaction with appearance as a 'normative discontent' (Rodin 1985, cited Rumsey and Harcourt 2005). In a survey of 2,100 adults in England, 61% of women and 35% of men reported concern about an aspect of their appearance (Harris and Carr 2001). Given the extent of such concerns, it is possible to underestimate the impact they may have and their ability to undermine quality of life (Pruzinsky 2004).

Body image has been defined as 'a loose mental representation of body shape, size and form which is influenced by a variety of historical, cultural and social, individual and biological factors which operate over varying time spans' (Slade 1994). However, Cash and Pruzinsky (2002) suggest that the term conveys the notion of a single image and propose the term *body experience* to convey the multifaceted nature of how we perceive and feel about our body and how it is intertwined with feelings about the self. Body experience is open to change (Pruzinsky 2004) and a rheumatic condition poses many challenges to a person's body experience.

When it is healthy, the body 'slips into the corporeal background and fades into the context of our lived experience' (Shilling 2005, p. 184). Its functioning is taken for granted, and we are often unaware of its presence. However, in the context of illness, the body comes to the fore (Pruzinsky 2004). We become conscious of its working and how other people may react to it.

Changes in appearance can have a significant negative impact on feelings of sexuality and attractiveness and on personal and sexual relationships (Gutweniger et al. 1999; Hill et al. 2003). Concerns about hand deformity have been identified as a factor associated with women seeking corrective hand surgery (Vamos et al. 1990). Studies of appearance concerns in people with rheumatic conditions report associations with anxiety and depression (Carr 1999; Jolly et al. 2008, 2011; Monaghan et al. 2007) which, in some instances, can lead to people withdrawing from social activities rather than risk confronting the potentially critical judgements of others (Rumsey 2002). There are a number of ways in which rheumatic conditions impact upon body experience (Table 13.2)

There are other more subtle ways in which the body is experienced differently. The boundaries of personal privacy may change if assistance is required with personal care:

> My carer is a 23-year-old girl. Now while she's excellent it was very very embarrassing at first when I was stood in the shower, you can imagine can't you? She is young enough to be my grand-daughter   (Robert OA).

The body becomes a focus for clinical examination which extends the boundaries of personal intimacy and requires people to engage with different perspectives of their body such as images derived from x-rays and scans. The boundaries of the natural body may be changed by the introduction of artificial joints and a new clinical language is acquired to describe the body which is not only confined to clinical encounters but is often used to convey information to friends, families and colleagues.

As suggested earlier, the link between the body and society is fundamental to any discussion on this topic in terms of how society shapes and informs how we feel about, understand and evaluate our body and the outward appearance we

Table 13.2 Examples of how rheumatic conditions impact upon body experience.

Examples of impact	Personal narrative
Deformities of hands, feet and spine	'It's your confidence, because when you are out in pubs or whatever and you are all hunched up, the way you walk and things like that, it does put people off. It does affect things like that so it affects your confidence' (Peter, AS)
Weight gain	'I weaned myself off prednisolone because my face went bigger and even now on my tummy its Prednisolone fat, you can tell, and my breasts are much bigger and I feel as if I'm pregnant sometimes. I have trousers I can't wear now because I've got this roll on my tummy and that's medicinal' (Shirley, RA)
Weight loss	'I lost it that fast, my bust completely went and my skin changed because of all the tablets and so you end up, for me, wrinkly around your bust and your tummy, so it isn't as if you've just lost weight gradually and you've kept some subtlety about it, so its spoilt it all' (Kate, RA)
Responding to disease exacerbations	'If I'm bad I tend to wear baggy clothes that aren't tight on my joints and I try to find soft cosy fabrics that are gentle. I need to wear things that I can get on the settee and curl up in and it doesn't matter if they get creased. I look for baggy things that I can move about in easily. Sometimes the effort of getting dressed in smart clothes is just too much' (Anne, RA)
Practical problems with dressing, styling hair and using of make-up	'All my clothes I had to give away and I bought things with elastic sides but I feel about 95 when I've got them on'. (Maureen, RA)
	'I've got very curly hair and you can see it's very straight now as I've had to have it cut very close to my head because I can't blow it. I can't pluck my eyebrows anymore either' (Shirley, RA)
Change in self-esteem	'I just feel a mess, that's all I can say, just a mess. My skin is more dry and thinner. I used to feel that I looked nice, everybody used to remark on how smart I was. But things changed. I can't wear nice shoes any more. I always used to wear a scarf and matching gloves, but I can't get gloves to fit any more. And so you end up looking for easier things to wear and I feel I'm turning into a mess' (Heather, RA)

strive to achieve. A person's appearance may become the focus of unwanted attention, something that strangers stare at which reinforces the feeling that the body does not meet the social ideals of beauty with which we are confronted (Lempp et al. 2006; Plach 2004).

I can see people looking at me because both of my feet point out and they look at me (Deborah RA).

As suggested by Rumsey and Harcourt (2005, p. 3), our physical appearance provides 'powerful cues for identity and recognition by others', and the negative judgements of others as discussed in Chapter 2 have the potential to become internalised (Charmaz 1983) and have a negative psychological impact (Thomas 1999).

Contemporary television programmes and numerous publications have demonstrated the positive impact that image management strategies can have on a person's appearance, self-confidence and feelings of self-worth. Whilst image consultancy requires specialist knowledge and expertise, informed conversations can take place in a clinical context which acknowledge the impact of rheumatic conditions upon this aspect of a person's life and signal a willingness to attempt to address such issues, potentially helping individuals to find a more positive way of thinking about and managing the impact of a changing body.

13.3   An introduction to strategies to increase confidence in personal presentation and clothing style

Personal appearance has a pervasive impact on our self-image and on the image we communicate to others, and clothing choice represents an effective and efficient means of controlling and managing the way we look (Damhorst 1990). Looking good and feeling good are inextricably linked:

> I like that feeling when you put something on because you can conquer the world if you feel right with what you've got on. With any woman if you get the right clothes you're fit to tackle anything (Pippa, RA).

People have a tendency to dwell on the negative rather than dressing to concentrate attention on their most flattering features. Understanding assets, and being able to focus and capitalise on them, builds confidence, alters self-perception and allows a greater feeling of 'normality'. The secret of successful dressing lies in buying and wearing clothes that reflect individual personality and enhance body shape and in choosing colours in harmony with skin, hair and eye tones.

Opening conversations

For someone struggling to feel good about their changing body there is something enormously cathartic in being able to express such feelings to a thoughtful and professional 'listening ear'. To ensure that incorrect assumptions are not made it is important to understand what matters to an individual. It is easy to assume that a person with highly visible deformities may be more distressed than a person with few visible signs of deformity when in fact the reverse may be true.

Enabling a person to voice their feelings, frustrations and difficulties may be an emotional experience as it may be the first time they have been allowed to fully express the impact that their condition has had on their self-perception. It is important to listen to, and fully acknowledge, frustrations and then to begin to move the focus from the negative to the positive by encouraging a positive assessment of 'best bits'. What are the features that deserve to be accentuated and appreciated and that an individual really likes and appreciates about themselves? It could be the eyes, smile, body shape, hair or posture.

Strategies

Helping people find practical solutions and things that work for them can create enthusiasm and an 'I can' rather than 'I can't' mentality, enabling them to enjoy and connect to the things they choose to wear. There are a number of strategies that can help people regain their confidence and feel more accepting of the visual effects of the disease.

Shifting the focus

By deliberately creating focal points the eye of the onlooker can be moved away from any challenge to a different part of the body. This can be helpful when no solution can be found to hiding a deformity or for detracting from a pair of orthopaedic shoes. The easiest way to create focal points is through the use of accessories; a pretty scarf, great brooch or interesting necklace will capture attention, particularly if it is in a colour that suits the wearer.

Using colour

Most people stick to safe colours and have very neutral wardrobes built around black, grey, beige and navy. However, an injection of colour can make a significant difference because wearing colours that work brings a healthy glow to the complexion and a feeling of vibrancy. Understanding the full range of colours that work for a particular combination of eye colour, hair colour and skin tone would involve a full colour consultation to which some people may be open. Alternatively, a person could be encouraged to think about the colours they love and get compliments for wearing and bring more of these into their wardrobe, particularly in tops and accessories. They can also work with the principle that 'like enhances like' and reflect their eye and hair colour in the clothing they buy.

Understanding body shape

Understanding the curves and lines of our bodies means that we can dress more easily and are better equipped to buy clothing that suits us. It is simple geometry; vertical lines lengthen and horizontal lines widen. Therefore, to appear taller and slimmer the eye needs to be kept moving vertically. Simple tips to appearing slimmer include:

- wearing garments with as many vertical lines as possible,
- using darker colours to cover a figure challenge,
- using fabrics that drape and do not cling,
- using matt not shiny fabrics and
- finding good, well-fitting underwear.

Hair and make-up

Hair and make-up can make a significant difference to the way women look and feel and are great morale boosters. A great haircut can bring modernity and make us look

10 years younger. Looking after and styling hair can be problematic for people with restricted arm movement and hand dexterity. A consultation with a good hairdresser, who understands the challenges a person faces, can lead to a stylish cut which is easy to care for and maintain. The same is true of make-up and, given the range of free advice from in-store make up counters, time can be spent experimenting with colour and products.

Shopping strategies

Shopping can be a challenge due to poor mobility, fatigue, inaccessible changing rooms, the need for assistance when trying on clothes and reliance upon others who may not share the same interest in shopping. People may also feel that their choices on the high street are compromised; they cannot buy 'normal' shoes, or dresses with zips, or pull on tights and a myriad of other challenges that have to be taken into account. Shopping habits can be adapted by:

- planning shopping trips in April and October when stores have the best stock and maximum choice,
- using pacing techniques to ensure that maximum energy is conserved for shopping with coffee stops and, if necessary, a planned rest at the end of the trip,
- if possible shopping early in the day, or early in the week, as shops are quieter and provide a better service. Late night shopping can also be less stressful than weekends,
- making sure clothes are not restrictive and feel comfortable standing and sitting,
- developing an understanding of shops that suit a person's budget, shape and personality and provides the level of service and access that is required and
- finding a good alterations tailor can make a big difference to changing fastenings to make them easier to manage.

Some people may opt to do more of their shopping via the internet. Whilst this can be a solitary experience, a friend could be invited to join in the session. However, the personal value of shopping, for some people, should also be acknowledged:

> I used to spend most Saturdays browsing in the shops looking at the latest fashions. Now I just pick something up as quickly as possible. It was one of my biggest passions and now I hate it (Peggy RA).

Developing a personal style

Shopping and buying the right clothes can be made easier by developing an understanding of personal style. To understand a personal style, a range of images a person loves can be pulled together to build a collage using pictures of garments, colours and interiors taken from magazines. Looking at the overall picture will help to understand style preference and clarify how these can be brought into wardrobes.

The strategies outlined serve as an introduction to how a person can be encouraged to address some of the image-related challenges they may face. As described earlier, for some people, investing in time with an image consultant can have a significant impact on their confidence, self-esteem and body experience.

13.4   The impact of rheumatic conditions on personal and sexual relationships

Sexuality encompasses sex, gender identities and roles, sexual orientation, eroticism, pleasure, intimacy and reproduction (WHO 2002). It is experienced and expressed through 'thoughts, fantasies, desires, beliefs, attitudes, values, behaviour, practices, roles and relationships' and is influenced by 'the interaction of biological, psychological, social, economic, political, cultural, ethical, legal, historical, religious and spiritual factors' (WHO 2002, p. 3). Therefore, it is important to recognise the multifaceted nature of sexuality.

Impact on personal relationships

Rheumatic conditions may impact negatively on personal as well as sexual relationships and both aspects of a person's relationship need to be explored. A negative impact on a sexual satisfaction does not necessarily equate with a negative impact on a relationship satisfaction. Yoshino and Uchida (1981) found that whilst participants in their study reported lower levels of sexual satisfaction, they reported higher levels of relationship satisfaction.

In studies undertaken with people with rheumatic conditions, associations have been made however between the level of adjustment within the relationship to the illness and levels of depression, disease progression and coping (Lanza et al. 1995; Mann and Dieppe 2006; Revenson and Majerovitz 1991). Mann and Dieppe (2006) identified three different responses to how couples dealt with RA within their relationship comprising: shared illness management, in which both partners were actively engaged with decisions relating to illness management; the ill partner in charge where the person with RA made autonomous decisions about their condition management; conflict over management group in which there was conflict about how the person with RA was managing their condition.

Whilst clinical attention often focuses on the needs of the person with the impairment, a survey of family members of people with RA highlighted the many ways in which RA impacts of partners and the need for healthcare professionals to consider the needs of partners alongside the person with RA (National Rheumatoid Arthritis Society 2012).

Clients not in relationships may experience increased difficulty in finding a partner due to the negative impact of the condition on their self-esteem, reduced engagement in social activities and concerns about disclosing their impairment.

Impact on sexual relationships

People with rheumatic conditions can experience reduced frequency of sexual intercourse and also reduced sexual satisfaction due to factors including pain and fatigue, limited mobility and dexterity, depression, reduced self-esteem and the effects of some medication (Cakar et al. 2007; Healey et al. 2009; Hill et al. 2003; Ryan 2008). Partners of people with long-term conditions can also experience an increase in demands as they assume more responsibility within the family or carryout extra tasks alongside providing support to their partner, all of which can impact upon sexual relationships (Gordon and Perrone 2004). Many people with rheumatic conditions report poor sleep due to pain and discomfort which can also result in couples sleeping in separate beds and in some instances separate rooms (Yoshino and Uchida 1981). Specific strategies that may be helpful in overcoming some of the difficulties people experience in engaging in sexual intercourse are provided in the Arthritis Research UK Booklet Sex and Arthritis (2010).

Addressing sexual relationships issues in practice

Whilst research evidence highlights the negative impact of rheumatic conditions on sexual relationship, studies undertaken with healthcare professionals show consistently that many healthcare professionals experience difficulty in addressing this aspect of peoples' lives in clinical practice (Ryan and Wylie 2005; Tristano 2009). Reasons for this include lack of confidence and expertise, lack of privacy and time (Ryan and Wylie 2005). There have been ongoing calls within the occupational therapy literature for occupational therapists to acknowledge sexual activity as a component of an holistic client-centred approach (Couldrick 1998, 2005; Sakellariou and Algardo 2006).

In light of the concerns expressed by healthcare professionals, the PLISSIT model (Anon 1976) offers an approach which enables therapists to address clients' needs to a level to which they, as healthcare professionals, feel confident and comfortable. The PLISSIT model (Box 13.2) comprises four levels of intervention with each level requiring greater knowledge and expertise.

Whilst healthcare professionals may feel that they are open to discussing sexual relationship issues this may not be clear to clients, and a negative cycle is entered in which professionals state that clients are reticent to discuss such issues as they are never raised and clients feel professionals are reticent as they never ask about them. In their work to develop an extended version of the PLISSIT model, Taylor and Davis (2006) highlighted the need for healthcare professionals to give permission at every stage of the process within the PLISSIT model not only by asking direct questions but by the availability of information in waiting areas or the inclusion of information, where relevant, in booklets and leaflets the department may produce which signals a willingness to engage with this topic.

> **Box 13.2   PLISSIT model of sexual counselling**
>
> **P (Permission)**
>
> This is the most basic level of intervention in which the topic of sexuality is introduced signalling a willingness to engage with this topic and encouraging a person to discuss concerns they may have.
>
> **LI (Limited Information)**
>
> At this level limited information is provided that is in direct reference to concerns mentioned earlier in the permission stage. It may be via factual information in pamphlets, booklets or other resources.
>
> **SS (Specific Suggestions)**
>
> This level requires greater knowledge and expertise as a more detailed sexual history is obtained to identify specific problems. Interventions suggested may relate to compensatory techniques, problem solving with the person and their partner about alternative sexual positions or the use of sex aids.
>
> **IT (Intensive Therapy)**
>
> This level of intervention requires formal training and will usually require a referral to a specialist service.

13.5   Conclusions

Whilst the clinical management of rheumatic conditions is predicated upon client-centred working located within a biopsychosocial model of practice, addressing the impact of these impairments upon a person's self-image and their personal and sexual relationships is an area of practice which is often neglected. Throughout this and preceding chapters, the links between self-concept, self-esteem, self-confidence and self-image have been highlighted consistently as has the influence these aspects of self exert on engagement in meaningful occupation roles and activities.

Resources

Books & Publications

Henderson V, Henshaw P (2010) *Colour Me Beautiful: Change Yours Truly, Look Change Your Life*. London: Hamlyn.

National Rheumatoid Arthritis Society (2012) *Family Matters. A Major UK Wide Survey on the Family Living with Rheumatoid Arthritis*. http://www.nras.org.uk/campaign/surveys/impact_on_the_family_survey_2012.aspx. Accessed on 12 November 2012.

Wan G (2008) *How to Look Good Naked. Shop for Your Shape and Look Amazing.* London: Harper Collins.

Woodall T, Constantine S, Matthews R (2002) *What Not to Wear.* London: W&N.

Websites

Arthritis Research UK Sex and Arthritis. www.arthritisresearchuk.org/arthritis-information/arthritis-and-daily-life/sex-and-arthritis.aspx. Accessed on 14 November 2012.

Relate provide both relationship counselling and sex therapy. www.relate.org.uk

Associations

The Association of Stylists and Image Professionals provides direct access to the services of personal stylists and image consultants through its website: www.asiplo don.com. Accessed on 14 November 2012.

The Federation of Image Professionals International supports, develops, promotes and regulates the image profession both in the United Kingdom and internationally: www.fipigroup.com. Accessed on 14 November 2012.

References

Anon J (1976) The PLISSIT model: A proposed conceptual scheme for the behavioural treatment of sexual problems. *Journal of Sex Education Therapy* 2:1–15.

Cakar E, Dincer U, Kiralp M, et al. (2007) Sexual problems in male ankylosing spondylitis patients: Relationship with functionality, disease activity, quality of life and emotional status. *Clinical Rheumatology* 26:1607–1631.

Carr A (1999) Beyond disability: Measuring the social and personal consequences of osteoarthritis. *Osteoarthritis Cartilage* 7:230–238.

Cash T, Pruzinsky T (eds.) (2002) *Body Image. A Handbook of Theory, Research and Clinical Practice.* New York: Guildford Press.

Charmaz C (1983) Loss of self: A fundamental form of suffering in the chronically ill. *Sociology of Health and Illness* 5:168–195.

Couldrick L (1998) Sexual issues: An area of concern for occupational therapists. *British Journal of Occupational Therapy* 61(11):493–496.

Couldrick (2005) Sexual expression and occupational therapy. *British Journal of Occupational Therapy* 68(7):315–318.

Cronin Mosley A (1986) *Psychosocial Components of Occupational Therapy.* New York: Raven Press.

Damhorst M (1990) In search of a common thread: Classifications of information communicated through dress. *Clothing and Textiles Research Journal* 8:1–12.

Devins G (2006) Psychologically meaningful activity, illness intrusiveness, and quality of life in rheumatic diseases. *Arthritis Care and Research* 55(2):172–174.

Devins GM, Edworthy SM, Guthrie NG, et al. (1992) Illness intrusiveness in rheumatoid arthritis: Differential impact on depressive symptoms over the adult lifespan. *Journal of Rheumatology* 19:709–715.

Gordon PA, Perrone KM (2004) When spouses become caregivers: Counselling implications for younger couples. *Journal of Rehabilitation* 70(2):27–31.

Gutweniger S, Kopp M, Mur E, et al. (1999) Body image of women with rheumatoid arthritis. *Clinical Experimental Rheumatology* 17(4):413–417.

Harris D, Carr A (2001) Prevalence of concern about physical appearance in the general population. *British Journal of Plastic Surgery* 54:223–226.

Healey E, Haywood K, Jordan K, et al. (2009) Ankylosing spondylitis and its impact on sexual relationships. *Rheumatology* 48:1378–1381.

Hill J, Bird H, Thorpe R (2003) Effects of rheumatoid arthritis on sexual activity and relationships. *Rheumatology* 44(2):280–286.

Jolly M, Brown C, Harris C, et al. (2008) Body image related quality of life in women with rheumatoid arthritis. *Arthritis & Rheumatism* 58(9 suppl):S279.

Jolly M, Pickard AS, Mikolaitis RA, et al. (2012) Body image in patients with systemic lupus erythematosus. *International Journal of Behavioral Medicine* 19(2):157–164.

Katz PP, Yelin EH (2001) Activity loss and the onset of depressive symptoms: Do some activities matter more than others? *Arthritis Rheumatism* 44:1194–1202.

Katz PP, Morris A, Yelin EH (2006) Prevalence and predictors of disability in valued life activities among individuals with rheumatoid arthritis. *Annals of Rheumatic Diseases* 65:763–769.

Lanza AF, Cameron AE, Revenson TA (1995) Perceptions of helpful and unhelpful support among married individuals with rheumatic diseases. *Psychology and Health* 10:449–462.

Lempp H, Scott D, Kingsley G (2006) The personal impact of rheumatoid arthritis on patient's identity: A qualitative study. *Chronic Illness* 2(2):109–120.

Mann C, Dieppe P (2006) Different Patterns of illness related interaction in couples coping with rheumatoid arthritis. *Arthritis Care and Research* 55(2):279–286.

Monaghan SM, Sharpe L, Denton F, et al. (2007) Relationships between appearance and psychological distress in rheumatic diseases. *Arthritis and Rheumatism* 57(2):303–300.

National Rheumatoid Arthritis Society (2012) *Family Matters. A Major UK Wide Survey on the Family Living with Rheumatoid Arthritis*. http://www.nras.org.uk/campaign/surveys/impact_on_the_family_survey_2012.aspx. Accessed on 12 November 2012.

Plach S, Stevene P, Moss V (2004) Corporeality: Women's experience of a body with rheumatoid arthritis. *Clinical Nursing Research* 13(2):137–155.

Pruzinsky T (2004) Enhancing quality of life in medical populations: A vision for body image assessment and rehabilitation as standards of care. *Body Image* 1:71–81.

Reinseth L, Espnes G (2007) Women with rheumatoid arthritis: Non-vocational activities and quality of life. *Scandinavian Journal of Occupational Therapy* 14:108–115.

Reinseth L, Till U, Kjeken I, et al. (2010) Performance in leisure-time physical activities and self-efficacy in females with rheumatoid arthritis. *Scandinavian Journal of Occupational Therapy* 18(3):210–218.

Revenson TA, Majerovitz SD (1991) The effects of chronic illness on the spouse: Social resources as stress buffers. *Arthritis Care Research* 4:63–72.

Rumsey N (2002) Body image and congenital conditions with visible differences. In: Cash TF, Pruzinsky T (eds.) *Body Image*. London: Guilford Press.

Rumsey N, Harcourt D (2005) *The Psychology of Appearance*. Maidenhead, UK: Open University Press.

Ryan S (2008) Assessing the effects of fibromyalgia on patient's sexual activity. *Nursing Standard* 23(2):35–41.

Ryan S, Wylie E (2005) An exploratory survey of the practice of rheumatology nurses addressing the sexuality of patients with RA. *Musculoskeletal Care* 3(1):44–52.

Sakellariou D, Algardo SS (2006) Sexuality and occupational therapy: Exploring the link. *British Journal of Occupational Therapy* 69(8):350–356.

Shilling C (2005) *The Body in Culture, Technology and Society*. London: Sage.

Slade P (1994) What is body image? *Behavioural Research and Therapy* 32(5):497–502.

Taylor B, Davis S (2006) Using the extended PLISSIT model to address sexual healthcare needs. *Nursing Standard* 21(11):35–40.

Thomas C (1999) *Female Forms*. Buckingham, UK: Open University Press.

Tristano AG (2009) The impact of rheumatic disease on sexual function. *Rheumatology International* 29(8):853–860.

Vamos M, White G, Caughey D (1990) Body image in rheumatoid arthritis: The relevance of hand appearance to desire for surgery. *British Journal of Medical Psychology* 63(3):267–277.

World Health Organization (2002) *Defining Sexual Health. Report of a Technical Consultation on Sexual Health 28–31 January, 2002 Geneva*. Geneva: World Health Organization, 2006.

Yoshino S, Uchida S (1981) Sexual problems of women with rheumatoid arthritis. *Archives of Physical Medicine and Rehabilitation* 62:122–123.

Index

Note: Page numbers in *italics* refer to Figures; those in **bold** to Tables.
